MEIOSIS

Edited by **Carol Bernstein**
and **Harris Bernstein**

Meiosis
http://dx.doi.org/10.5772/56972
Edited by Carol Bernstein and Harris Bernstein

Contributors
Takashi Ohyama, Érica Duarte-Silva, Angela Maria Hauck Duarte Silva, Adriano Silvério, Elvira Hoerandl, Philip Bell, Carol Bernstein

Published by InTech
Janeza Trdine 9, 51000 Rijeka, Croatia

Publishing Process Manager Ana Pantar
Technical Editor InTech DTP team
Cover InTech Design team

Additional hard copies can be obtained from orders@intechopen.com

Meiosis, Edited by Carol Bernstein and Harris Bernstein
p. cm.
ISBN 978-953-51-1197-9

For EU product safety concerns:
IN TECH d.o.o., Prolaz Marije Krucifikse Kozulić 3, 51000 Rijeka, Croatia,
info@intechopen.com or visit our website at intechopen.com.

Meet the editor

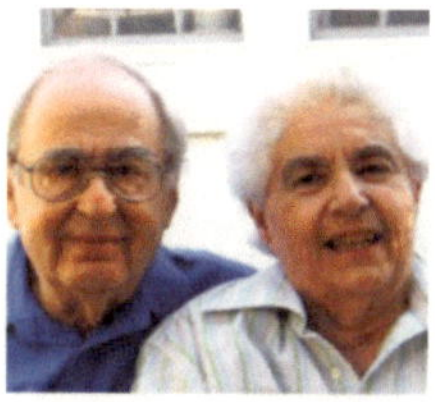

Carol and Harris Bernstein received their PhDs in Genetics from the University of California (Davis) and from the California Institute of Technology, respectively. They subsequently met and got married while at Yale in 1962. They were faculty members at the University of Arizona College of Medicine for 43 years, retiring in 2011. Their research interests focus on DNA damage and its underlying role in sex, aging and in the early steps of initiation and progression to cancer. In their research, they have used organisms including bacteriophage T4, Neurospora crassa, Schizosaccharomyces pombe and mice, as well as human cells and tissues. They have authored (jointly and singly) more than 140 scientific publications, including articles in major peer reviewed journals, book chapters and invited reviews.

Contents

Preface

Meiosis is the key process underlying sexual reproduction in eukaryotes, occurring in single-celled eukaryotes and in most multicellular eukaryotes including animals and most plants. Thus meiosis is of considerable interest, both at the scientific level and at the level of natural human curiosity about sexual reproduction. Improved understanding of important aspects of meiosis has emerged in recent years and major questions are starting to be answered, such as "How does meiosis occur at the molecular level?", "How did meiosis and sex arise during evolution?", "What is the major adaptive function of meiosis and sex?". In addition, changing perspectives on meiosis and sex have led to the question: "How should meiosis be taught?" .

The first chapter in this book reviews a number of recent studies indicating that double-stranded DNA molecules can distinguish "self" from "non-self" and consequently can undergo self-assembly in a pair-wise manner even in a solution of heterogeneous double-stranded DNA species. These studies used experimental approaches involving electrophoretic analysis and atomic force microscopy, analysis of liquid-crystalline aggregates, and a technique involving parallel single molecule magnetic tweezers applied to isolated double-stranded DNA. In addition, this chapter reviewed evidence that this type of selective association between homologous DNA molecules also applies to nucleosomes. Self-assembly of homologous double-stranded DNA molecules and homologous nucleosomes is a central molecular step in meiosis.

The next three chapters are concerned with the origin and function of meiosis. The first two of these chapters emphasize that central enzymatic features of meiosis were already present in the prokaryotic ancestors of eukaryotes. One of these chapters went further, indicating that the prokaryotic ancestor was likely able to undergo transformation, a process of DNA transfer between individual bacteria. In transformation, the central proteins catalyzing this process are homologous to proteins with similar functions in meiosis. The other of the first two chapters emphasizes the triggering role of DNA damage in initiating meiosis as well as the purging role of deleterious mutations in diploid-haploid cycles. The major function of meiosis, dealt with extensively in these two chapters, is DNA repair of unavoidable damages in germ line DNA. Especially discussed is the need for meiosis-provided homologous recombinational repair of double-strand breaks and cross-links in the germ line. Both chapters discuss difficulties with earlier proposals that the main selective advantage of meiosis is the long term benefit of producing genetic variation. The third chapter in this section points out characteristics of the eukaryotic cell (such as coding for mRNA capping enzymes and phage-type RNA polymerases in mitochondria) that could have been derived from symbiogenic complex viruses. These characteristics led the author to propose a viral eukaryogenesis theory. By this theory, meiosis is derived from the processes by which a postulated viral ancestor of the nucleus infected new hosts.

The last chapter of the book presents a practical approach to teaching meiosis and gives examples of how a low cost program can be set up. This program will allow students to understand the general processes employed by different types of plants that undergo meiosis. It emphasizes gross morphology and aspects of morphology that can be observed with a hand lens or under a microscope.

Carol Bernstein and Harris Bernstein
Department of Cellular and Molecular Medicine
University of Arizona, USA

Section 1

Molecular Basis of Meiosis

Chapter 1

Intrinsic Homology-Sensing and Assembling Property of Chromatin Fiber

Jun-ichi Nishikawa, Yasutoshi Shimooka and Takashi Ohyama

Additional information is available at the end of the chapter

http://dx.doi.org/10.5772/56548

1. Introduction

The first meiotic prophase is divided into five sequential stages, referred to as *leptotene, zygotene, pachytene, diplotene* and *diakinesis*. Chromosome pairing is initiated during the late *leptotene* and early *zygotene*. As the stage progresses, the four chromatids are arranged and form two distinct pairs of sister chromatids, and the two chromatids in each pair are tightly aligned along their entire lengths. The synaptonemal complex (SC) is fully formed at the *pachytene* stage. Although such morphological changes in chromosomes and the mechanism of recombination have been well studied, we do not still understand how each chromosome recognizes and approaches its matching mate or homologue and the mechanism by which it interacts and pairs with its homologue. Regarding the latter phenomenon, double-stranded (ds) DNA has long been considered to have the ability to distinguish self and non-self. Indeed, this property of DNA was predicted about 60 years ago (Jehle, 1950; Yos *et al.*, 1957) and was directly demonstrated a half-decade ago, when dsDNA molecules were proved to have sequence-sensing and self-assembly properties (Inoue *et al.*, 2007). In the following two years, other studies describing the presence of such properties in DNA were reported (Baldwin *et al.*, 2008; Danilowicz *et al.*, 2009). A more recent study has revealed that nucleosomes retain this DNA sensing property and can self-assemble (Nishikawa and Ohyama, 2013). In this chapter, we define the self-association of the same dsDNA molecules as DNA self-assembly and that of nucleosomes with identical DNA as nucleosome self-assembly. And, we will discuss the recent findings on DNA self-assembly and nucleosome self-assembly and their relationships, as putatively significant mechanisms in the early stage in meiosis.

2. Self-assembly in biological systems

Self-assembly is the autonomous organization of constituents into higher-order structures or assemblages, in which disordered pre-existing components form organized architectures as a consequence of specific, local interactions among the components, without external intervention. This phenomenon is widely found in the natural world, and is a fundamental mechanism in biological systems (Whitesides and Grzybowski, 2002). A characteristic of biological self-assembly is the variety and complexity of the functions of the resulting structures (Kushner, 1969; Perham, 1975). We see such examples in lipid bilayer formation, base pairing, protein folding, protein-protein interactions, including the formation of quaternary structures, protein-nucleic acid interactions, flagella formation from flagellin, actin assembly, microtubule and microfibril formation, and virus, organ and cell assembly (Kushner, 1969; Whitesides and Grzybowski, 2002; Mueller *et al.*, 1962; Watson and Crick, 1953; Oosawa and Asakura, 1975; Asakura, 1968; Horváth *et al.*, 1949; Miki-Noumura and Mori, 1972; Fraser *et al.*, 1976; Fraenkel-Conrat and Williams, 1955). Generally, self-assembly occurs by the tendency of a system to move toward the state of minimum free energy, and the assemblages are the result of the thermodynamic equilibrium, which is determined by various conditions, including temperature, pH, pressure, the concentrations and/or chemical potentials of various molecules and ions (Oosawa and Asakura, 1975) and London-van der Waals forces (Jehle, 1963).

3. DNA can sense homology and self-assemble

The possibility of a nucleotide sequence-dependent, selective interaction between dsDNA fragments was first studied theoretically (Kornyshev and Leikin, 2001). The following scenario was depicted: sequence-dependent twist modulation leads to axial variation of the local helical pitch, which allows an electrostatically favorable alignment of two DNA fragments; as the result, only DNA with homologous sequences can have negatively charged strands facing positively charged grooves over a large juxtaposition length, and nonhomologous sequences cannot align well because they require higher energy for juxtaposition. In another model, proposed over 40 years ago, the homology recognition is based on non-Watson-Crick hydrogen bond interactions occurring between bases in the major or minor grooves (McGavin, 1971). In still another model, proposed over 50 years ago, homology recognition is based on correlations in the fluctuating polarizations of nearby identical molecules (the London-van der Waals force) (Yos *et al.*, 1957).

The first experimental evidence proving that DNA can sense homology and self-assemble was obtained in 2007 (Inoue *et al.*, 2007). Electrophoretic analyses of thirteen different dsDNA molecules with ~100 - ~800 bp lengths and an atomic force microscopy (AFM) analysis revealed that in a solution composed of heterogeneous DNA species, DNA molecules preferentially interact with the molecules bearing an identical sequence and length, and they can form assemblages (Fig. 1A). This phenomenon efficiently occurs in the presence of physiological concentrations of Mg^{2+} ions, usually several mM. Nanomolar DNA concentrations also seem

http://dx.doi.org/10.5772/56548

to be a prerequisite for the stable formation of self-assemblages. Interestingly, curved DNA and DNA with an A-form-like conformation also exhibited the self-assembling property. Thus, this phenomenon is not specific to the usual B-form DNA, but seems to be general for all kinds of dsDNA.

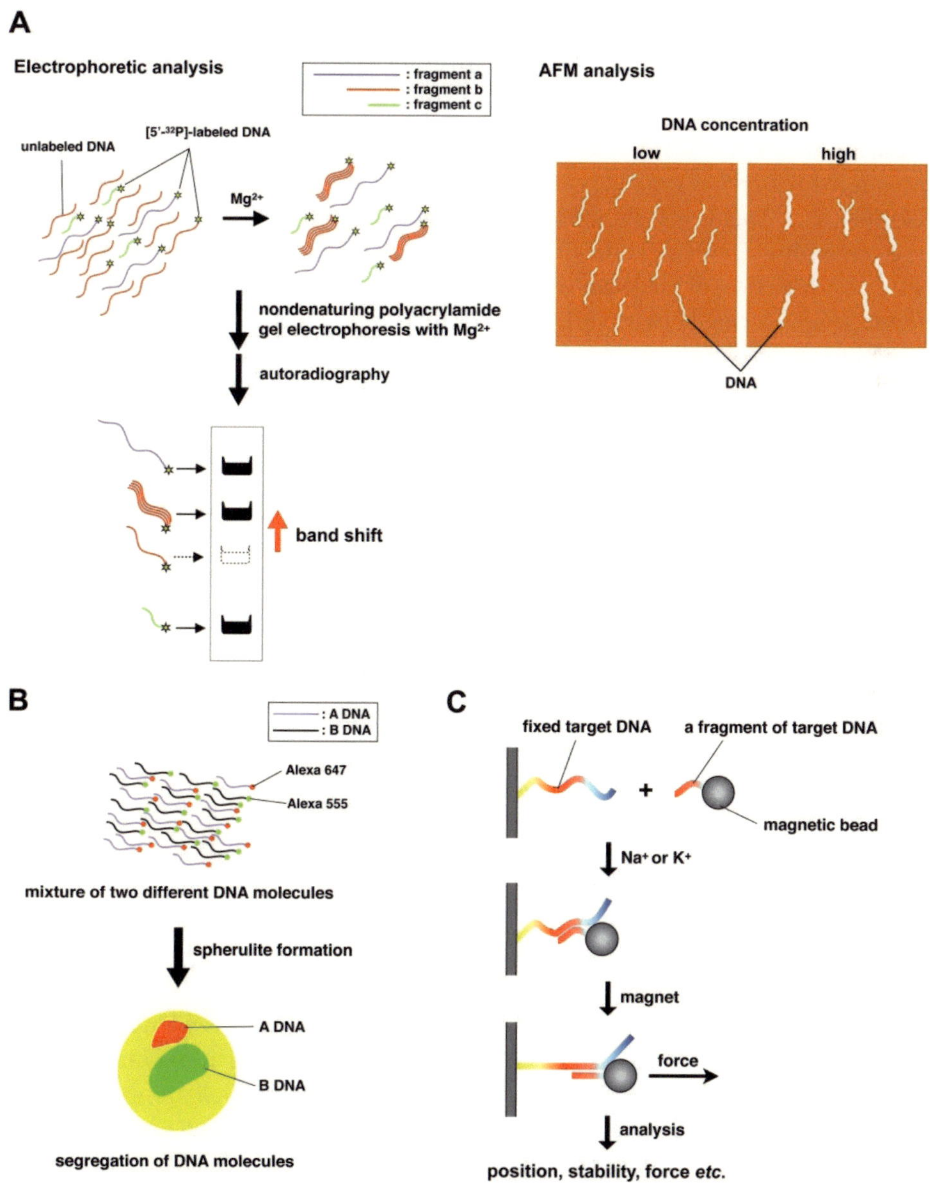

Figure 1. Three different experimental approaches proved intrinsic homology-sensing and assembling property of dsDNA. (A) Electrophoretic and AFM analyses (Inoue *et al.*, 2007). (B) Spherulite analysis (Baldwin *et al.*, 2008). (C) Parallel single molecule magnetic tweezers-based assay (Danilowicz *et al.*, 2009).

In 2008 (Baldwin *et al.*, 2008), another experimental approach confirmed this homology-sensing and pairing ability of dsDNA. In this approach, 5′-amine-modified-DNAs with ~300 bp lengths were labeled with either Alexa Fluor 555, a green fluorescent tag, or Alexa Fluor 647, a far-red fluorescent tag, condensed into aggregates, mounted on microscope slides, equilibrated for two weeks, and subjected to a confocal microscopy analysis. Interestingly, segregation of the two kinds of DNA was observed within each spherulite (discrete liquid-crystalline aggregate) (Fig. 1B). Although the experimental conditions seemed to be far from *in vivo* conditions (extremely high concentrations of NaCl (> 0.5 M) and DNA were used to generate spherulites), this study succeeded in extracting a hidden property of dsDNA.

In 2009, using phage λ DNA and a parallel single molecule magnetic tweezers-based assay, an experiment further confirmed the presence of homologous dsDNA pairing (Danilowicz *et al.*, 2009) (Fig. 1C). This study showed that pairing can occur even in the absence of divalent cations or crowding agents. Specifically, the pairing occurred in the presence of more than 50 mM Na^+ or K^+ (the effect of the latter was generally smaller than that of the former). In 10 mM Na^+, homologous pairing between λ DNA and its 5 kb fragment was not detected. However, significant homologous pairing was detected between the two at 10 mM Mg^{2+}. Although a 10 mM Mg^{2+} concentration may be slightly higher than the *in vivo* concentration (Terasaki and Rubin, 1985), the essence of this finding was the same as that in the report by Inoue *et al.* (2007). Furthermore, the detected pairs were stable against thermal forces (up to ~50°C) and shear forces up to 10 pN. Homologous pairing was detected at 1-3 nM DNA, which was also consistent with the report by Inoue *et al.* (2007).

In conclusion, the three above-mentioned studies proved that dsDNA has homology-sensing ability and can self-assemble, but the mechanism underlying the phenomenon remains enigmatic. The next issue to be discussed is whether nucleosomes, the fundamental units of chromatin (Luger *et al.*, 1997), have sequence-dependent self and non-self discrimination properties. Regarding this, to our knowledge, no report has ever been presented. Before moving on to this subject, let's review the structures of chromatin and nucleosomes.

4. Nucleosomes, the fundamental units of chromatin

Chromatin provides the structural basis for all nuclear events involving DNA, such as replication, transcription, repair and recombination (Ransom *et al.*, 2010; Svejstrup, 2010; Weake and Workman, 2010). The main building block of chromatin is the nucleosome (Oudet *et al.*, 1975), the core of which consists of 146-147 bp of DNA and a histone octamer of two each of the four core histones H2A, H2B, H3, and H4. The DNA is wrapped around the histones to form 1.65-1.67 turns of left-handed supercoils (Davey *et al.*, 2002; Luger *et al.*, 1997). The main body of chromatin fibers has nucleosome cores, core-connecting linker DNAs (Felsenfeld and Groudine, 2003; Simpson, 1978), and a specific complement of associated proteins such as the linker histone H1, localized at DNA entry and exit sites protruding from the nucleosome core, and architectural proteins (McBryant *et al.*, 2006, 2010; Thoma *et al.*, 1979). The simplest form of chromatin is the "beads-on-a-string" structures (10 nm fibers) formed by nucleosomes and

http://dx.doi.org/10.5772/56548

linker DNAs (Thoma *et al.*, 1979). The secondary packaging level of chromatin is thought to be 30 nm fibers, which have been observed in thin sections of intact cells and whole mount preparations (Igo-Kemenes *et al.*, 1982; Kornberg, 1977; Richmond and Widom, 2000; and references therein). High ionic strength and the presence of linker histones can fold 10 nm fibers into 30 nm fibers *in vitro* (Huynh *et al.*, 2005). However, the structures and higher order organization remain uncertain and various models have been proposed (Finch and Klug, 1976; Robinson *et al.*, 2006; Schalch *et al.*, 2005; Williams *et al.*, 1986; Woodcock *et al.*, 1984). Furthermore, recently a considerable controversy has arisen regarding the existence of 30 nm fibers *in vivo* (Eltsov, 2008; Fussner *et al.*, 2011; Nishino *et al.*, 2012).

5. Nucleosomes can self-assemble

Our recent study (Nishikawa and Ohyama, 2013) strongly suggested that nucleosomes have sequence-dependent self and non-self discrimination properties, and can self-assemble. We constructed oligonucleosomes using DNA octamers or tetramers and histone cores. Each of the original DNA fragments had 177 or 209 base pairs and contained a clone of *Xenopus* 5S rDNA nucleosome positioning sequence or those of artificial DNA sequences designated 601 and 603. The latter two clones were selected to contain strong nucleosome positioning sequences with high affinity for histone octamers (Lowary and Widom, 1998). We used various arrangements of these nucleosomes. The resulting oligonucleosomes were then subjected to AFM observations. Interestingly, we found that the nucleosomes with identical sequences tended to associate with each other in the oligonucleosomes. However, the movement of nucleosomes in a nucleosomal array was restricted in this system. Therefore, to determine whether the same kind of association occurs in a system free from such a structural restriction, we also examined nucleosome-nucleosome interactions using bead-fixed mononucleosomes and Alexa 555-labeled mononucleosomes. In this system, association was monitored as the increase of fluorescence intensity on the beads. This assay clearly showed that associations between the same nucleosome species were preferred over those between different species. Based on the topological aspects, the contact points in the association seem to reside on the core histone proteins (Fig. 2). It was speculated that the mechanisms underlying the self-assembly of homologous dsDNAs and those mediating the self-assembly of homologous nucleosomes may be different (Nishikawa and Ohyama, 2013).

6. DNA self-assembly and nucleosome self-assembly may be key players in presynaptic alignment

The pairing of homologous chromosomes begins during the late *leptotene* and early *zygotene* phases of meiosis. At first, homologous chromosomes are brought into close vicinity by some mechanism. In fission yeast, noncoding RNA seems to play this role. A recent study showed that even when homologous chromosomes are apart from each other, they can interact with assistance from noncoding RNA in fission yeast (Ding *et al.*, 2012). Transcriptional machinery

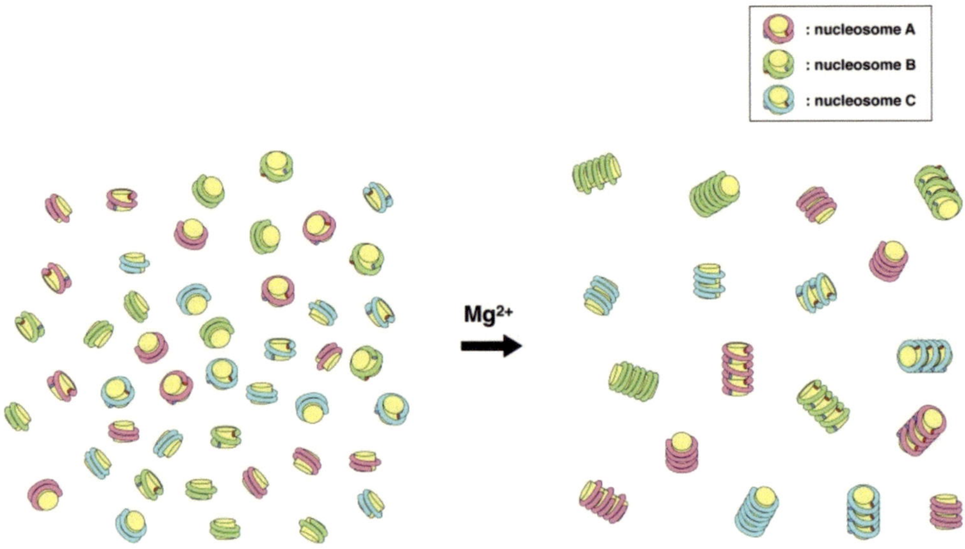

Figure 2. Nucleosomes have sequence-dependent self and non-self discrimination properties. Our study suggested that the contact points in the association of nucleosomes reside on the core histone proteins (Nishikawa and Ohyama, 2013).

proteins, cohesin, insulator or Polycomb proteins, may also play a similar role (Cook, 1997; McKee, 2004; Blumenstiel *et al.*, 2008). Subsequently, homologous chromosomes recognize each other securely and align (pair), in preparation for synapsis. This stage is referred to as presynaptic alignment, and it may involve weak, homologous, paranemic DNA/DNA interactions (Stack and Anderson, 2001). The finding of the self-assembling property of DNA seems to substantiate this hypothesis. However, "paranemic DNA/DNA interactions" should be reconceptualized as "paranemic chromatin fiber/chromatin fiber interactions", because the DNA sequence-dependent self-assembling property of nucleosomes has also been proved to exist. In this discussion, a chromatin fiber is the 10 nm fiber, or the beads-on-a-string chromatin fiber.

In mammals, plants and fungi, the recombination pathway is often functionally interdigitated with presynaptic alignments and synapsis. Namely, in some organisms, meiotic double-stranded break (DSB) formation and recombination are required for these processes (Zickler, 2006; Zetka, 2009). On the other hand, in *Drosophila* and *C. elegans*, these processes proceed in the absence of DSBs and recombination (McKim *et al.*, 1998; Dernburg *et al.* 1998; Zetka, 2009). Thus, DNA self-assembly and nucleosome self-assembly may be the essential mechanism of at least presynaptic alignment of the latter group (Fig. 3). Furthermore, they may also function in SC formation.

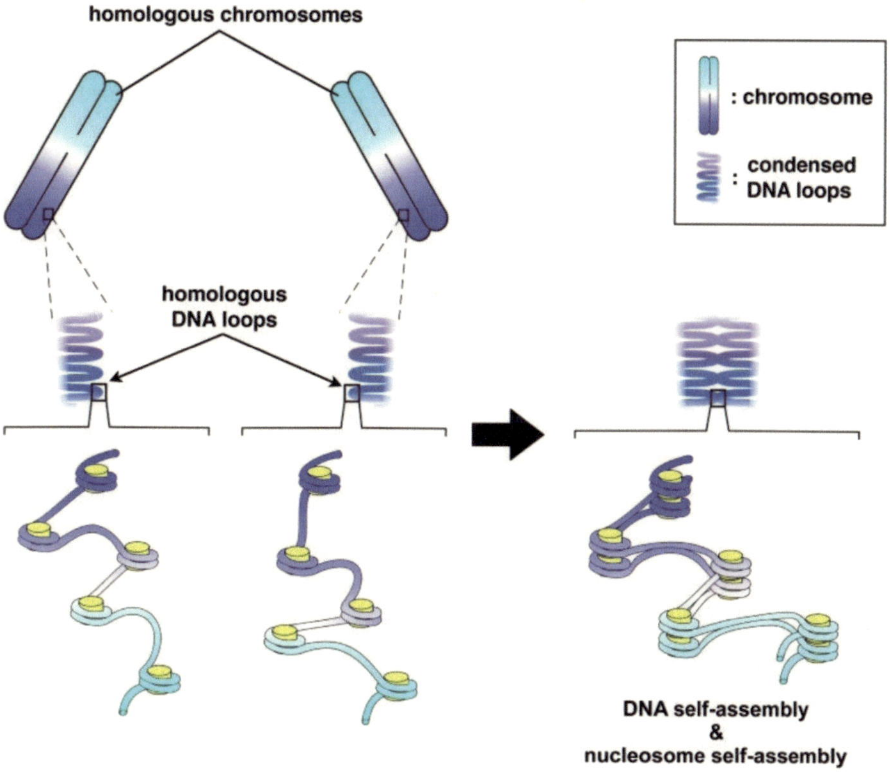

Figure 3. Schematic representation of DNA self-assembly and nucleosome self-assembly in paired homologous chromosomes.

7. Conclusion

In this chapter, we have described that both DNA and nucleosomes have sequence-dependent self and non-self discrimination properties, and can self-assemble. These properties of DNA and nucleosomes seem to be the key mediators of presynaptic alignment in some organisms. We hypothesize that the attractive force facilitating DNA self-assembly and nucleosome self-assembly is widely employed in many biological processes, including not only meiotic chromosome pairing but also somatic chromosome pairing, such as polytene chromosome formation in *Diptera*, transvection and other similar phenomena.

Acknowledgements

We acknowledge the support of the Ministry of Education, Culture, Sports, Science & Technology - Japan (MEXT) to T.O.

Author details

Jun-ichi Nishikawa[1], Yasutoshi Shimooka[2] and Takashi Ohyama[2*]

*Address all correspondence to: ohyama@waseda.jp

1 Department of Biology, Faculty of Education and Integrated Arts and Sciences, Waseda University, Shinjuku-ku, Tokyo, Japan

2 Integrative Bioscience and Biomedical Engineering, Graduate School of Science and Engineering, Waseda University, Shinjuku-ku, Tokyo, Japan

References

[1] Asakura, S. (1968). A kinetic study of in vitro polymerization of flagellin. J. Mol. Biol. , 35, 237-239.

[2] Baldwin, G. S, Brooks, N. J, Robson, R. E, Wynveen, A, Goldar, A, Leikin, S, Seddon, J. M, & Kornyshev, A. A. (2008). DNA double helices recognize mutual sequence homology in a protein free environment. J. Phys. Chem. B , 112, 1060-1064.

[3] Blumenstiel, J. P, Fu, R, Theurkauf, W. E, & Hawley, R. S. (2008). Components of the RNAi machinery that mediate long-distance chromosomal associations are dispensable for meiotic and early somatic homolog pairing in Drosophila melanogaster. Genetics , 180, 1355-1365.

[4] Cook, P. R. (1997). The transcriptional basis of chromosome pairing. J. Cell Sci. , 110, 1033-1040.

[5] Danilowicz, C, Lee, C. H, Kim, K, Hatch, K, Coljee, V. W, Kleckner, N, & Prentiss, M. (2009). Single molecule detection of direct, homologous, DNA/DNA pairing. Proc. Natl. Acad. Sci. USA , 106, 19824-19829.

[6] Davey, C. A, Sargent, D. F, Luger, K, Maeder, A. W, & Richmond, T. J. (2002). Solvent mediated interactions in the structure of the nucleosome core particle at 1.9 Å resolution. J. Mol. Biol. , 319, 1097-1113.

[7] Dernburg, A. F, Mcdonald, K, Moulder, G, Barstead, R, Dresser, M, & Villeneuve, A. M. (1998). Meiotic recombination in *C. elegans* initiates by a conserved mechanism and is dispensable for homologous chromosome synapsis. Cell , 94, 387-398.

[8] Ding, D. Q, Okamasa, K, Yamane, M, Tsutsumi, C, Haraguchi, T, Yamamoto, M, & Hiraoka, Y. (2012). Meiosis-specific noncoding RNA mediates robust pairing of homologous chromosomes in meiosis. Science , 336, 732-736.

[9] Eltsov, M. MacLellan, K.M., Maeshima, K., Frangakis, A.S. and Dubochet, J. ((2008). Analysis of cryo-electron microscopy images does not support the existence of 30-nm

chromatin fibers in mitotic chromosomes in situ. Proc. Natl. Acad. Sci. USA , 105, 19732-19737.

[10] Felsenfeld, G, & Groudine, M. (2003). Controlling the double helix. Nature , 421, 448-453.

[11] Finch, J. T, & Klug, A. (1976). Solenoidal model for superstructure in chromatin. Proc. Natl. Acad. Sci. USA , 73, 1897-1901.

[12] Fraenkel-conrat, H, & Williams, R. C. (1955). Reconstitution of active tobacco mosaic virus from its inactive protein and nucleic acid components. Proc. Natl. Acad. Sci. USA , 41, 690-698.

[13] Fraser, R. D. MacRae, T.P. and Suzuki, E. ((1976). Structure of the alpha-keratin microfibril. J. Mol. Biol. , 108, 435-452.

[14] Fussner, E, Ching, R. W, & Bazett-jones, D. P. (2011). Living without 30 nm chromatin fibers. Trends Biochem. Sci. , 36, 1-6.

[15] Horváth, I, Király, C, & Szerb, J. (1949). Action of cardiac glycosides on the polymerization of actin. Nature 164, 792.

[16] Huynh, V. A, Robinson, P. J. J, & Rhodes, D. (2005). A method for the *in vitro* reconstitution of a defined "30 nm" chromatin fibre containing stoichiometric amounts of the linker histone. J. Mol. Biol. , 345, 957-968.

[17] Igo-kemenes, T, Hörz, W, & Zachau, H. G. (1982). Chromatin. Annu. Rev. Biochem. , 51, 89-121.

[18] Inoue, S, Sugiyama, S, Travers, A. A, & Ohyama, T. (2007). Self-assembly of double-stranded DNA molecules at nanomolar concentrations. Biochemistry , 46, 164-171.

[19] Jehle, H. (1950). Specificity of Interaction Between Identical Molecules. Proc. Natl. Acad. Sci. USA , 36, 238-246.

[20] Jehle, H. (1963). Intermolecular forces and biological specificity. Proc. Natl. Acad. Sci. USA , 50, 516-524.

[21] Kornberg, R. D. (1977). Structure of chromatin. Annu. Rev. Biochem. , 46, 931-954.

[22] Kornyshev, A. A, & Leikin, S. (2001). Sequence recognition in the pairing of DNA duplexes. Phys. Rev. Lett. , 86, 3666-3669.

[23] Kushner, D. J. (1969). Self-assembly of biological structures. Bacteriol. Rev. , 33, 302-345.

[24] Lowary, P. T, & Widom, J. (1998). New DNA sequence rules for high affinity binding to histone octamer and sequence-directed nucleosome positioning. J. Mol. Biol. , 276, 19-42.

[25] Luger, K, Mader, A. W, Richmond, R. K, Sargent, D. F, & Richmond, T. J. (1997). Crystal structure of the nucleosome core particle at 2.8 Å resolution. Nature , 389, 251-260.

[26] Mcbryant, S. J, Adams, V. H, & Hansen, J. C. (2006). Chromatin architectural proteins. Chromosome Res. , 14, 39-51.

[27] Mcbryant, S. J, Lu, X, & Hansen, J. C. (2010). Multifunctionality of the linker histones: an emerging role for protein-protein interactions. Cell Res. , 20, 519-528.

[28] Mcgavin, S. (1971). Models of specifically paired like (homologous) nucleic acid structures. J. Mol. Biol. , 55, 293-298.

[29] Mckee, B. D. (2004). Homologous pairing and chromosome dynamics in meiosis and mitosis. Biochim. Biophys. Acta , 1677, 165-180.

[30] Mckim, K. S, Green-marroquin, B. L, Sekelsky, J. J, Chin, G, Steinberg, C, Khodosh, R, & Hawley, R. S. (1998). Meiotic synapsis in the absence of recombination. Science , 279, 876-878.

[31] Miki-noumura, T, & Mori, H. (1972). Polymerization of tubulin: the linear polymer and its side-by-side aggregates. J. Mechanochem. Cell Motil. , 1, 175-188.

[32] Mueller, P, Rudin, D. O, Tien, H. T, & Wescott, W. C. (1962). Reconstitution of cell membrane structure in vitro and its transformation into an excitable system. Nature , 194, 979-980.

[33] Nishikawa, J, & Ohyama, T. (2013). Selective association between nucleosomes with identical DNA sequences. Nucleic Acids Res. , 41, 1544-1554.

[34] Nishino, Y, Eltsov, M, Joti, Y, Ito, K, Takata, H, Takahashi, Y, Hihara, S, Frangakis, A. S, Imamoto, N, Ishikawa, T, & Maeshima, K. (2012). Human mitotic chromosomes consist predominantly of irregularly folded nucleosome fibres without a 30-nm chromatin structure. EMBO J. , 31, 1644-1653.

[35] Oosawa, F, & Asakura, S. (1975). Thermodynamics of the Polymerization of Protein (London: Academic Press).

[36] Oudet, P, Gross-bellard, M, & Chambon, P. (1975). Electron microscopic and biochemical evidence that chromatin structure is a repeating unit. Cell , 4, 281-300.

[37] Perham, R. N. (1975). Self-assembly of biological macromolecules. Philos. Trans. R. Soc. Lond. B , 272, 123-136.

[38] Ransom, M, Dennehey, B. K, & Tyler, J. K. (2010). Chaperoning histones during DNA replication and repair. Cell , 140, 183-195.

[39] Richmond, T. J, & Widom, J. (2000). Nucleosome and chromatin structure. In Chromatin Structure and Gene Expression, S.C.R. Elgin, and J.L. Workman, eds. (New York: Oxford University Press) , 1-23.

http://dx.doi.org/10.5772/56548

[40] Robinson, P. J. J, Fairall, L, Huynh, V. A. T, & Rhodes, D. (2006). EM measurements define the dimensions of the "30-nm" chromatin fiber: Evidence for a compact, interdigitated structure. Proc. Natl. Acad. Sci. USA , 103, 6506-6511.

[41] Schalch, T, Duda, S, Sargent, D. F, & Richmond, T. J. (2005). X-ray structure of a tetranucleosome and its implications for the chromatin fibre. Nature , 436, 138-141.

[42] Simpson, R. T. (1978). Structure of the chromatosome, a chromatin particle containing 160 base pairs of DNA and all the histones. Biochemistry , 17, 5524-5531.

[43] Stack, S. M, & Anderson, L. K. (2001). A model for chromosome structure during the mitotic and meiotic cell cycles. Chromosome Res. , 9, 175-198.

[44] Svejstrup, J. Q. (2010). The interface between transcription and mechanisms maintaining genome integrity. Trends Biochem. Sci. , 35, 333-338.

[45] Terasaki, M, & Rubin, H. (1985). Evidence that intracellular magnesium is present in cells at a regulatory concentration for protein synthesis. Proc. Natl. Acad. Sci. USA , 82, 7324-7326.

[46] Thoma, F, Koller, T. H, & Klug, A. (1979). Involvement of histone H1 in the organization of the nucleosome and of the salt-dependent superstructures of chromatin. J. Cell Biol. , 83, 403-427.

[47] Watson, J. D, & Crick, F. H. C. (1953). Molecular structure of nucleic acids: a structure for deoxyribose nucleic acid. Nature , 171, 737-738.

[48] Weake, V. M, & Workman, J. L. (2010). Inducible gene expression: diverse regulatory mechanisms. Nat. Rev. Genet. , 11, 426-437.

[49] Whitesides, G. M, & Grzybowski, B. (2002). Self-assembly at all scales. Science , 295, 2418-2421.

[50] Williams, S. P, Athey, B. D, Muglia, L. J, Schappe, R. S, Gough, A. H, & Langmore, J. P. (1986). Chromatin fibers are left-handed double helices with diameter and mass per unit length that depend on linker length. Biophys. J. , 49, 233-248.

[51] Woodcock, C. L. F, Frado, L. L. Y, & Rattner, J. B. (1984). The higher-order structure of chromatin: evidence for a helical ribbon arrangement. J. Cell Biol. , 99, 42-52.

[52] Yos, J. M, Bade, W. L, & Jehle, H. (1957). Specificity of the London-Eisenschitz Wang force. Proc. Natl. Acad. Sci. USA , 43, 341-346.

[53] Zetka, M. (2009). Homologue pairing, recombination and segregation in *Caenorhabditis elegans*. In Meiosis (Genome Dynamics R. Benavente, and J.-N. Volff, eds. (Basel: Karger) , 5, 43-55.

[54] Zickler, D. (2006). From early homologue recognition to synaptonemal complex formation. Chromosoma , 115, 158-174.

Section 2

Origin and Function of Meiosis

Chapter 2

Meiosis and the Paradox of Sex in Nature

Elvira Hörandl

Additional information is available at the end of the chapter

http://dx.doi.org/10.5772/56542

1. Introduction

The paradox of sex is still enigmatic and regarded as a major unresolved problem in evolutionary biology [1]. Sex is here understood as a process of organisms in which the genomes of two nuclei are brought together in a common cytoplasm to produce progeny which may then contain reassorted portions of the parental genomes. In eukaryotes, sex involves meiosis-mixis-cycles and is tied to reproduction. The prevalence of sexual reproduction in eukaryotes is striking because of the obvious high costs of sex [2]: first, recombination during meiosis breaks up beneficial gene combinations; associated with these processes are the risks of errors and mismatches during pairing of homologous chromosomes, plus the time needed for meiosis. The second cost is mixis, which requires two parental individuals for conducting fertilization, merging of cells and genomes. A couple of secondary costs are associated to mixis: mate searching, mate finding, costs of sexual selection, competition for mating partners, and finally physical contacts. The alternative, asexual reproduction without meiosis-mixis cycles, potentially avoids these costs; [3,4]. Paradoxically, rather few eukaryotes conduct asexual reproduction: less than 1% of species of animals and seed plants and 10% of ferns reproduce via asexuality, in fungi about 20%; only in protists obligate asexuality occurs more regularly in many phyla [5]. And, when eukaryotes shift to asexuality, they do not abandon sex completely, but often just modify the sexual meiosis-mixis cycle in various ways [6-8].

Meiosis, in fact, is the key process of sexual reproduction in eukaryotes, as it is the only shared and conserved feature of sex in eukaryotes. Meiosis originated early in eukaryotes, perhaps together with mitosis [9]. The cost of sex, thus, primarily applies to eukaryotes. Prokaryotes have less complex chromosomes, no meiosis, and thus they do not have a comparable cost. Mixis and syngamy, the second part of sexual reproduction, vary a lot in different eukaryote groups. Basically, two parental individuals are needed to conduct mixis, karyogamy and syngamy. Many evolutionary biologists put a lot of emphasis on the cost of "males", as male individuals do not produce offspring; asexual animals are thus expected to produce higher quantities of offspring than sexual ones. In animals, where separate sexes are the rule (ie. male and female individuals), the cost of males is regarded as a major problem [3,4]. However, many groups of eukaryotes do not produce "males" – most land plants are hermaphrodites in the sense that they have male and female organs on the same individual, either within one flower as in angiosperms (hermaphroditism) or in different flower-like structures on the same individual as in most gymnosperms, or on the prothallium of many ferns (monoecy). In hermaphrodites, the cost of sex is significantly reduced to the cost of producing male organs [10]. Many protists and algae even reproduce via isogamy and do not develop gender differentiation. Many fungi have dozens of different mating types, that is, genetically different hyphens, which equals to dozens of "genders". There is no general cost of males in eukaryotes, and the group-specific "cost of males" is a side aspect in the paradox of sex discussion.

Meiosis, in contrast, is the shared feature for eukaryotic sex. In fact, the problem of maintenance of sex can be largely referred to the question: "What is meiosis good for?" About 20 major hypotheses have been proposed to explain the paradox of sex, and three main theories attempt to explain the function of meiosis (see [11], for detailed review): 1) Meiotic sex is the mechanism for creating recombination and thus new gene combinations in the offspring, which would increase the evolutionary and adaptive potential of genetically variable offspring; 2) Meiosis is a restoration tool for promoting the integrity of nuclear DNA, by repairing DNA double strand breaks (DSB), by eliminating deleterious mutations, and by repair of epigenetic damage; 3) Meiosis is a phylogenetically conserved feature which cannot be eliminated because of the ancestral fixation of meiosis-mixis-cycles. None of these theories provide an all-inclusive answer for the paradox of sex [11-12]. These theories are not a priori exclusive, but may have combinational values.

Traditionally, sex has been seen as advantageous due to the effects of recombination during meiosis, a process which generates genetic variance in the offspring. Genetic variation can provide an adaptive benefit in changing environments [13-14]. Further, recombination exposes deleterious mutations to purifying selection. Selection against less fit mutants could help to purge deleterious mutations from the genome [15-16]. However, it was already recognized in the 1980s that these benefits do not sufficiently explain the high costs of obligate and regular sexual reproduction [17]. Selection can act against recombination, and recombination does not necessarily result in beneficial new gene combinations and traits [1]. Recombination is further an investment into an uncertain future. Many evolutionary biologists have pointed out that sex must be foresighted to make beneficial new gene combinations. But, evolution is blind and cannot have foresight. Individuals conducting sex gain no immediate advantage, and there is no benefit to the mating partners bearing all the costs of mate searching and recognition as well as the risks of sex. Some animals, such as many insects and fishes, even die directly after sexual reproduction. The selective forces to act on variable offspring do not provide benefits to the parents. That is, creating variation in the offspring is only a group advantage, but no individual advantage, which weakens the efficiency of selection for maintenance of sex [11].

These theoretical problems were largely recognized by evolutionary biologists already in the 1980s [17]. Several modifications have been proposed, but the key problem of recombination-based models remains: the benefit of recombination is context-dependent, but in many

http://dx.doi.org/10.5772/56542

eukaryotic organisms, sex is not at all context-dependent but obligatory. Recombination thus might be rather not the cause but a consequence of sex [12]. In this book chapter I will expand my recently proposed combinational theory for maintenance of sex [12] which suggests a combinational effect of DNA restoration mechanisms during meiosis as the major function of sex. DNA restoration is beneficial in any ecological context, and it provides a benefit for each offspring generation. However, this function of meiosis must be understood in a context of evolutionary history, eukaryotic metabolism and its inherent chemistry of life, in particular redox chemical reactions. First I will review some basic features of oxidative stress during aerobic respiration and photosynthesis, and the DNA damages caused by ROS. Second, I will review the current knowledge on evolution of meiosis as an homologous recombinational DNA repair mechanism. Third, I will discuss the evolution and function of meiosis proteins. Fourth, a hypothesis on the function of segregation and reductional division at meiosis will be discussed. Finally I will provide some suggestions for further studies to obtain more support for this hypothesis.

2. The origin of eukaryotic life, oxidative stress and DNA damage

Oxidative stress and DNA damage. Carol and Harris Bernstein [18-20] and coworkers were the first to propose a consistent hypothesis that crossing over at meiosis might have evolved as a repair mechanism of oxidative double strand DNA damage. Their ideas stemmed from observations that, in fact, meiosis is not at all optimized to create new gene combinations, as Holliday junctions can be resolved with and without cross-over. The frequencies of non-crossovers were shown to be higher than those of cross-overs, but only the latter create new gene combinations in flanking regions, which is most important for recombination. The idea emerged that meiosis could be a repair mechanism of DNA double strand breaks [18], for which a homologous chromosome is needed as template. Later, this idea was linked up to oxidative DNA damage [19-20]. However, since many other DNA repair mechanisms exist, and since permanent diploidy would also serve for DNA repair, the theory was not broadly accepted by evolutionary biologists [11]. It is useful to discuss this theory in view of evolutionary history, which was first attempted by Lynn Margulis [21].

The origin of the eukaryotic cell via endosymbiosis [21] is meanwhile a well-established theory; the inclusion of prokaryotic endosymbionts, which later became cell organelles, i.e. the mitochondria and, in plants, the plastids, were key innovations for eukaryotic metabolism as they allowed for aerobic respiration and photosynthesis, respectively. However, both aerobic respiration and photosynthesis are major sources of reactive oxygen species (ROS). Triplet oxygen, $^3O_2$, is not highly reactive but this is not the case for its radicals, which are formed by accidental one-electron transfers and its electronically excited state singlet oxygen [22], $^1O_2$. Especially the hydroxyl radical ($OH^\bullet$) and, to a lesser extent, the superoxide anion radical ($O_2^{\bullet-}$) cause many kinds of damages. By contrast, hydrogen peroxide (H_2O_2) is more stable, but also an oxidizing agent, and can be reduced to $OH^\bullet$ in the Fenton reaction in the presence of transition metal catalysts, such as iron or copper:

$H_2O_2 {}_+ Fe^{2+} \rightarrow OH^{\bullet} + OH^{-} + Fe^{3+}$

Photosynthesis is an old mechanism, invented by cyanobacteria, and probably evolved between 3.8 and 3.5 billion years ago. The basic chemical machinery of photosynthesis likely evolved out of defense mechanisms against UV-induced photochemical radicals, in a time before the development of a protective ozone layer. Early cyanobacteria probably used hydrogen sulfide (H_2S) as an electron source for an anoxygenic photosynthesis, which is only driven by photosystem I (PSI). As H_2S resources were depleted, mutants arose which combined PSI with PSII activity, which provided sufficient energy to facilitate the utilization of water as an electron source [23-24]. Another hypothesis explains the evolution of photosynthesis from the presence of hydrogen peroxide, H_2O_2, which was formed by UV irradiation (due to the lacking ozone layer); hydrogen peroxide can also serve as an electron source for photosynthesis but provides only two electrons per molecule [25]. Modern photosynthesis uses the energy of light to oxidize water (H_2O) as an electron source to generate chemical energy in the form of ATP; this energy is used to reduce carbon dioxide (CO_2) to sugars. The oxygenic photosynthesis, as we know it today, enabled organisms to produce organic compounds like sugars from atmospheric CO_2 much more efficiently. Oxygen was released into the atmosphere and hydrosphere as a gaseous waste product, simplified as:

$CO_2 + 2\,H_2O \rightarrow \langle CH_2O \rangle + H_2O + O_2$

The rise of oxygen concentrations in the atmosphere was initially slow, probably because oxygen was initially bound by metals, mainly iron, available in rocks and minerals. In the presence of oxygen, soluble ferrous iron (Fe^{2+}) is oxidized to insoluble rust (ferric iron, Fe^{3+}). Only between 2.2 and 2 billion years ago, the earth's atmosphere started to enrich in molecular oxygen released from the oxygenic photosynthesis of cyanobacteria; around 1.8 billion years ago the O_2 in the atmosphere reached 5-18% of the present level [26-27]. Around 1 billion years ago, the ozone layer formed from the release of oxygen in the atmosphere, protecting organisms from UV light. From this time onwards, the threats from UV irradiation for life have been reduced, but the ability to use oxygen and to cope with its high reactivity became a major evolutionary constraint for life on earth.

In modern green plants, photosynthesis during the light period is the major source of free oxygen radicals. Normally, the electron flow from the excited photosystem I is directed to NADP, which is reduced to NADPH. It then enters the Calvin cycle and reduces the final electron acceptor, CO_2. Transfer of excitation energy from excited chlorophylls to oxygen in the light-harvesting complexes leads to the formation of $^1O_2$ and $O_2^{\bullet -}$, which can be further converted to H_2O_2 and $OH^{\bullet}$. The production of ROS is enhanced by strong light and also by deceleration of the Calvin cycle [28]. In the dark period, most oxygen radicals are produced by mitochondria [29].

Aerobic respiration basically is an oxidative breakdown of organic molecules for gaining energy in the form of ATP equivalents, and, for this purpose, is a magnitude more efficient than anaerobic respiration. The reduction of oxygen provides the largest free energy release per electron transfer among all elements of the periodic system [27]. Anaerobic respiration uses sulfur, methane or hydrogen as electron acceptors. These sources were probably depleted in the early history of life, and may have been only locally abundant (e.g. sulfur may be locally concentrated around volcanoes, fumaroles etc.). By contrast, aerobic respiration can use dispersed atmospheric oxygen as the final electron acceptor. Oxygen respiration may have evolved in facultatively aerobic / anaerobic organisms, such as alpha-proteobacteria [30]. This second major invention was a major precondition for the origins of eukaryotes, because it allowed for an improved energy gain from food and substantial increase of growth and body size [27]. However, the price for this metabolic innovation was coping with oxygen radicals in the vital organelles *inside* the cells.

$$4\,e^{-} + 4\,H^{+} + O_2 \rightarrow 2\,H_2O$$

This transfer of four electrons to oxygen is controlled by the mitochondrial electron-transport chain but accidentally one-electron transfer may occur:

$$O_2 + e^{-} \rightarrow O_2^{\bullet -}$$

The mitochondrial electron-transport chain is perhaps the most important source of reactive oxygen species in animal cells [22, 31]. $O_2^{\bullet -}$ is transformed into H_2O_2 by enzymes such as superoxide dismutase (SOD). H_2O_2 is relatively stable, but membrane-permeable and can diffuse into the cytosol. When H_2O_2 is not removed by the antioxidant defense systems, such as ascorbic acid, hydroxyl radicals ($OH^{\bullet}$) can be generated through the metal-catalyzed Fenton reaction (see above). Moreover, oxygen may not only generate oxygen radicals, but also reactive nitrogen species (reviewed by [22]).

The electron transfers during respiration and photosynthesis basically occur in the membranes of mitochondria and plastids, respectively. The more stable H_2O_2 can potentially penetrate into the nucleus. In summary, aerobic respiration and the presence of oxygen in the cell created a new and continuous source of free radicals adding a new major *endogenous* threat of DNA damage. In anoxic periods, DNA damage was mostly caused exogenously by photosensitization of light exposed tissues. An excited photo-reactive compound can excite molecular oxygen into singlet $^1O_2$, which is much more easily reduced to $O_2^{\bullet -}$ than $^3O_2$ [32]. As previously described, superoxide anion radical can lead to the formation of hydroxyl radicals in the presence of catalytic transition metals. This new endogenous source of ROS, however, endangered the cell itself and is countered by an elaborate antioxidant defense system comprised of ascorbic acid, glutathione, and a complex enzyme machinery guaranteeing the regeneration of these reducing agents in attempts to maintain a redox homeostasis, which is vital for cell survival.

Oxygen radicals and DNA damage. Free radicals react readily with DNA, and the majority of oxidative damages occur in nuclear DNA [19]. Under the presence of oxygen, peroxyl radicals are formed by addition of molecular oxygen to DNA base or sugar radicals, which in turn may undergo complex reactions. For instance, thymine may react with $OH^{\bullet}$ at the C5–C6 double bond to form thymine glycol [33]. Thymine glycol is known to be a quite frequent source of DNA damage and blocks DNA replication and transcription [19]. This is just one of the many reactions and products of free radicals with DNA, which have been reviewed comprehensively elsewhere [22,33,34]. Hydroxyl radicals can cause not only single, but tandem lesions of purine bases [35]. An important feature of free radicals is that single initiation events have the potential to generate multiple reactions and multiple peroxide molecules by complex chain reactions [22]. Most importantly, free radicals may destroy the DNA 2-deoxyribose sugar. The highly reactive DNA sugar radicals may lead to the formation of altered sugars which may consequently lead to strand breaks at the sugar-phosphate backbone of DNA [33]. Free radicals are also involved in the formation of DNA-protein crosslinks, in which one DNA radical and one protein radical are involved [33].

As previously mentioned, various mechanisms have evolved in eukaryotes to deal with the toxicity of oxygen radicals. For instance, the superoxide dismutase enzymes (SODs) remove superoxide by catalyzing a redox reaction to form H_2O_2 and O_2. Catalases are the most important H_2O_2-removal systems in various eukaryotic organisms. Halliwell [22] gives a survey of the various antioxidant mechanisms in plants and animals; however, these systems are not 100% perfect. Moreover, reactive oxygen species may also have beneficial effects, such as defense mechanisms against pathogens, and regulation of cellular processes by influencing phosphorylation [22]. In plants, reactive oxygen species produced by photosynthesis may even be involved in regulation of gene expression and cell to cell signaling [36]. For these reasons, reactive oxygen species are never completely scavenged, but even may be produced on purpose [37]. When the balance of reactive oxygen species and antioxidants becomes shifted towards an excess of ROS, then increasing oxidative stress may lead to a damaging downward loop process, finally resulting in damage of DNA. Excessive DNA damage either halts the cell cycle to initiate repair, or ends in apoptosis [22].

With aerobic respiration and photosynthesis, eukaryotes were forced into the "oxygen paradox:" a highly efficient metabolism, but producing a continuous, internal source of damaging agents inside cells. Oxygen respiration was crucial for the evolution of high energy gain, and therefore complexity and multicellularity of eukaryotes. For its benefits, it is reasonable that oxygen respiration was maintained by selection in eukaryotes despite its detrimental side-effects. Because of the benefits of oxygen respiration, natural selection should rather favor improved repair mechanism of oxidative damages than abandoning oxygen respiration. The same principal may hold true for photosynthesis. Therefore, it is likely that enzymatic DNA repair mechanisms inherited from prokaryotes have been maintained and improved in eukaryotes. Eukaryotic cells have to repair DNA continuously and multiple DNA repair mechanism are known [34].

3. Homologous recombinational DNA repair of oxidative damage

Recombinational repair. It is well established that recombinational repair of DNA is the most efficient and accurate mechanism for repairing DNA double strand damages [38-40]. Many repair mechanisms deal with single strand-breaks that represent the most common type of DNA lesions. Single strand damages use the other strand as a template for repair. However, if a replication fork encounters a single strand break in its template, then a double-strand break might be the consequence [34]. For the evolution of meiosis, the repair mechanisms of double

http://dx.doi.org/10.5772/56542

strand breaks are of major interest. Double strand breaks can be repaired by non-homologous repair such as end-joining as well, but this mechanism is prone to error and a source of insertions, because ligation of free ends often leaves flaps of DNA strands [34,38,41]. Homologous recombinational repair, by contrast, requires a second, homologous, undamaged chromosome. This can be either a sister chromatid or a chromatid from another homologous chromosome.

The early eukaryotes were probably unicellular, haploid organisms. The increased internal oxidative damage introduced by cellular respiration (in plants, mainly by photosynthesis) in early eukaryotes required an elaborate mechanism for repair of double strand damage of the nuclear genome: this is only provided by homologous recombinational repair. Mitotic repair via the sister chromatid can cope with internal DNA damage as well, but this mechanism has two limitations: First, a sister chromatid is needed which is not available in the G1 and S phase of the cell cycle. DNA damage at these stages rather triggers regulated arrest mechanisms, so that replication is blocked [34]. That means that mitotic homologous recombinational repair is only available during growth, either in cell colonies or in tissues. DNA damage increases in postmitotic tissues of multicellular organisms [19], likely because homologous repair during mitosis is not available any more. Other repair mechanisms are mutagenic and lead to a slow but steady accumulation of mutations in somatic cells of multicellular organisms. The second limitation of mitotic repair is the need for resources, as each round of mitotic cell division requires DNA and protein synthesis to produce viable daughter cells. Hence, two rounds of mitosis with two synthesis phases are required to result in four daughter cells, while meiosis produces four daughter cells with just one synthesis phase. If resources are depleted, then organisms have problems to continue mitotic cell divisions because homologous recombinational repair with sister chromatids is too costly. If at the same time oxidative damage is accumulating, then the organism would have to conduct non-recombinational repair to avoid cell death. Non-recombinational repair, however, is prone to errors and mutational changes.

For a eukaryotic, unicellular organism, non-recombinational repair would not allow for continuity and integrity of the genome. Therefore, the early haploid protists had to find a way out of this dilemma: the most efficient way to survive oxidative stress under unfavorable growth conditions was to merge with another individual and to use the homologous chromosome set of the mating partner for DNA recombinational repair. Mixis provides a second, homologous chromosome – one that may also be damaged to some extent, but at sites different from damages in the other paired chromosome. This merging had a two-fold advantage: first, DNA double strand breaks can be efficiently repaired by homologous recombination with a second template; second, four daughter cells can be produced with only one synthesis phase. For a unicellular protist, mixis followed by meiosis was an efficient way to avoid cell death in unfavorable environments.

Meiosis and DNA repair. Initially, double strand breaks caused by oxidative damage could have been the primary trigger for the onset of meiosis. Carol Bernstein [20] summarized the main requirements for oxidative damage being a selective pressure for the maintenance of meiosis as a DNA repair mechanism in eukaryotes. To maintain meiosis by selection for DNA repair caused by oxidative damage, the following conditions must be fulfilled: (1) Oxidative damage is deleterious to cell function; (2) oxidative damage accumulates in somatic cells; (3) oxidative damage should be repairable by recombinational repair during meiosis; (4) the mechanisms of recombination enzymes should be more adapted to DNA repair than to simple random genetic exchange. Current evidence supports all these predictions.

1. Oxidative damage is deleterious to cell function. Since oxygen radicals are highly reactive, they basically attack each organic molecule around, damaging membrane lipids, proteins, and DNA. The immediate consequences of DNA damage are transcription termination, interruption of replication, and reduced cell survival. Oxidative stress leads to release of transition metal ions which may catalyze free-radical reactions. Oxidative stress further increases levels of free Ca^{2+}, which may result in a permeability transition of mitochondria. It is established that excessive oxidative stress initiates cell death, i.e., apoptosis [22]. Dead cells may further release metal ions and other toxic compounds to the neighboring cells, increasing the damage.

2. Oxidative damage accumulates in somatic cells of multicellular organisms. Oxidative DNA damages in somatic cells are by far the most frequent ones in mammals. Around 130,000 endogenous damages of DNA occur per cell per day for rats, whereby 86,000 are due to oxidative damage [20]. Oxidative damage may accumulate in the following way: free radicals first cause mutations of mitochondrial (mt) DNA, which, in turn, affects structure and function of mt proteins. Defective mt-encoded proteins result consequently in defective electron transport, which increases frequencies of free radicals. Free radicals finally diffuse into the cytosol and cause damage in the whole cell, including nuclear damage. Oxidative damage occurs first in the DNA of mitochondria and chloroplasts, and later also affects nuclear DNA [42]. This downward loop process continuously increases effects of oxidative damage and is seen as a main cause of somatic degeneration and ageing in multicellular organisms. Somatic cells accumulate oxidative damage as their fate is anyway death. In the germline, oxidative stress may even be a major cause for the evolution of anisogamy and gender differentiation. In complex multicellular organisms, the female germline is usually kept in a stage with inactive pro-mitochondria to protect from oxidative damage of aerobic respiration; the mitochondria are therefore inherited maternally. ATP is provided by cells surrounding the oocytes. The male sperm cells, in contrast, are being produced continuously, with meiosis as a repair mechanism. The spermatocytes are motile in many eukaryotes, and their active mitochondria already suffer from oxidative damage as a consequence of motility; thus, only the nucleus is transmitted to the zygote, while the mitochondria of male gametes are usually not inherited [42]. This division-of labor principle guarantees undamaged mitochondria for the offspring. Maternal inheritance of plastids in plants may follow similar principles.

3. Oxidative damage is repairable by recombinational repair. If the original function of meiosis is to repair DNA damages, then oxidative damage must be reparable by homologous recombination. Most damages affect just single strands of DNA, and repair can be conducted by the complementary strand which stores redundant sequence information for re-synthesis. Double-strand breaks and DNA cross-links cannot be easily repaired this

way, and these damages require information from a second, undamaged homologous DNA molecule by recombinational repair [20].

If oxidative damage is a trigger for recombinational repair at meiosis, then meiosis should be inducible by oxidative stress. The idea is supported by experimental work of the Bernstein group on the yeast *Schizosaccharomyces pombe* [20]. Strains of this free living, haploid, facultatively sexual-asexual organism have been treated with H_2O_2 in an adequate nitrogen medium, and the ratios of spores to colony forming units have been measured. The ratio was 4-18fold higher than for cells that were not exposed to H_2O_2. Most strikingly, this increase of sporulation was also observed in a nitrogen-rich medium, which means that starvation is not a primary cause for sporulation. DNA damage induces meiosis even under favorable nutritious conditions, which means that (1) recombination is here not conducted to create new gene combinations in the offspring that may adapt better to the changed environmental situation; (2) for excessive DNA damage, mitotic repair is insufficient. These experiments demonstrate that oxidative stress can induce meiosis in this yeast. Fission yeast can serve as a model for a simple, unicellular, haplontic protist that forms a diploid zygote only under stress conditions.

In the facultative sexual / asexual green alga *Volvox carteri*, sex is a response to increased levels of stress [43-44]. In this species, heat stress causes the production of a 30kDA glycoproteic inducer (SI). This inducer stimulates the gonidia to produce egg- or sperm bearing sexual spheroids. The fusion of gametes results in the formation of a desiccation-resistant, over wintering zygospore, which germinates and undergoes meiosis when favourable conditions return in the next spring. In this organism, sexual development in the gonidia is triggered by an approximately two-fold increase of reactive oxygen species after heat stress, and it could be demonstrated that ROS actually activate two sex genes, the SI gene and the clone B gene. These genes must have been ROS activated, because catalases decreased their transcript level [43-44]. The formation of the zygospore is likely a response to increased oxidative stress, and meiosis is the mechanism of recombinational DNA repair before the next haploid generation is formed. Nedelcu et al. [43, 44] suggest that sex might be one alternative as a stress response besides cell-cycle arrest and apoptosis.

Further support for an evolution of meiosis as a response to DNA lesions is available from research on the protist *Tetrahymena* by the group of Josef Loidl [45]. *Tetrahymena* has a micronucleus capable of meiosis, and a "vegetative" macronucleus. Elongation of the micronucleus and formation of a so-called "crescent" is the beginning of meiosis and normally induced by the enzyme spo11. However, micronucleus elongation can be also induced by DNA damaging agents such as UV irradiation and chemicals, even in spo11 deficient-mutants. These findings suggest that DNA damage is actually the trigger for spo11 activity. Interestingly, meiosis can be induced even by lesions other than DNA breaks, which is probably mediated by a phosphokinase signal transduction pathway [45]. These findings support the hypothesis that meiosis evolved in early eukaryotes as a response to several kinds of DNA damage.

The damaging effects of ROS on DNA, and their sex-inducing effects, strongly support a hypothesis that the need for a highly efficient DNA repair mechanism was the selective force for the evolution of homologous chromosome pairing and formation of chiasmata and crossovers at meiosis.

4. The mechanisms of recombination enzymes should be more adapted to repair than to simple random genetic exchange. This was one of the key arguments of Bernstein et al. [18] for the hypothesis that meiosis evolved as a repair mechanism of DNA. In the majority of cases, recombination does not result in an exchange of flanking regions of the DNA strands, which are much larger than the recombined regions and would efficiently create new gene combinations. Meiosis is consequently not optimized for creating genetic diversity, but for recombinational repair. Recent findings on the evolution of meiosis proteins strongly support this idea.

4. The evolution and function of meiosis proteins revisited

Many enzymatic activities related to DNA repair existed in prokaryotes before the evolution of eukaryotes with their onset of meiosis, namely, the cut- and paste activities of topoisomerases, recombinational break repair activities, including RecA-type recombinases, mismatch repair activities, and the clustering of telomeres and their dragging across the nuclear envelope [46]. Arguments in favour of a predisposition to meiosis in prokaryotes are that the core genes involved in meiosis have homologs in prokaryotes [46-48]. For instance, Rad51, which is found in almost all major groups of eukaryotes, is homologous to RecA in bacteria and RadA in Archaea [47-48]. RecA type recombinases are present in all living cells, and act in eukaryotes during mitotic recombinational repair [46]. Recombinational repair is already crucial for bacteria for viability despite the availability of other repair mechanisms. However, recombinational repair in circular DNA bears the danger of inversions or split of the ring-like genome into parts, while linear chromosomes can be more easily repaired [49]. Research in the last decade has elucidated the functions of eukaryotic proteins involved in meiosis [38-39,46-48,50]: Many of them are not specific for meiosis, but also act at recombinational repair at mitosis, such the mismatch repair proteins (Mlh1-3, Msh 2, 6). Some proteins represent a "core" meiosis-specific subset: Hop1, Hop2 and Mnd1 are responsible for homologous pairing; Spo11 is associated with double-strand breaks at the beginning of meiotic recombination; REC8 is a meiosis-specific paralog of mitotic RAD21, that is involved in sister chromatid cohesion; RAD52 mobilizes single-strand DNA for homology search. Rad51 is a key protein for heteroduplex formation. It is highly conserved among eukaryotes and acts during mitotic repair, and interacts with the meiosis-specific Dmc1 protein for strand exchange during meiosis. Rad51 is homologous to the bacterial RecA recombinase, an important repair enzyme. During meiosis, Rad51 is assisted by its meiosis-specific paralog Dmc1 for the formation of Holliday-junctions. Dmc1 is required for the formation of inter-homolog joint molecule recombination. Rad51 and Dmc1 probably work together promoting meiotic recombination events. The function of the Rad51 paralogs is not yet clear, but they likely play a role in homologous recombination. Heteroduplex DNA and crossing over is processed by mismatch-related repair proteins (Msh4, Msh5). Brca2 plays an early role in homologous recombination and very likely controls the formation of the Rad51/single-strand DNA nucleofilament. The MRX complex is a tripartite complex, with Mre1 and Rad50 being strongly conserved among eukaryotes. Both proteins are probably involved in double-strand end processing. The MRX complex probably has multiple roles during meiosis.

The key proteins of meiosis have obviously originated out of repair proteins, and still act during meiosis. They provide for successful pairing, Holliday junction formation, homologous repair and resolution of Holliday junctions. *Arabidopsis*-mutants with defects in these key recombination proteins show chromosomal instability during meiosis, which is frequently associated with sterility [38]. The question is – is modern meiosis also a consequence of oxidative stress, or is the protein activity at meiosis a cause of DSBs?

In extant organisms, DSBs are thought to be generated "on purpose" by the meiosis-specific Spo11 orthologs [41]. This seems to be a paradox – why should intact DNA strands be broken only to be repaired afterwards again? Double strand breaks belong to the most serious lesions of DNA, and different solutions exist to resolve Holliday junctions (HJ): only some of them lead to cross-over, ie. an exchange of genes on the two homologous chromatids, which potentially creates new beneficial gene combinations. HJ dissolution, but also some forms of double strand break repair do NOT result in an exchange of flanking regions (which would have efficiently created new gene combinations) [38]. HJ are thus not efficient processes for creating new gene combinations, which questions whether the function of spo11 is to make "programmed" breaks. In many extant organisms, spo11 is present together with DSBs and caps the cleaved DNA strand ends. The function of spo11 must be understood from a perspective of evolutionary history and its chemistry. Spo11 has evolved from archaeal topoisomerase VI via several gene duplications [48]. All eukaryotic lineages were preceded by the origin of Spo11 from topoisomerase VI homologs, which means that spo11 originated before eukaryotes diversified.

The evolution of Spo11 suggests that this protein most probably originally did *not* have a function of "creating" double strand breaks [48]. First, a gene duplication generated spo11-3, which is not meiosis-specific. Spo11-3 is present in protists, the choanoflagellate *Monosiga*, and in plants; in other eukaryotic lineages, this ortholog was probably secondarily lost. The function of this basic spo11-3 homolog is still not well understood, but it is *not* involved in meiotic recombination. Later on, gene duplications separated spo11-3 from the meiosis-specific homolog spo11-2, which is again found mainly in protists and plants, and is phylogenetically sister to spo11-1 which is found in protists, plants, animals and fungi. Only the meiosis-specific orthologs act during meiosis in animals, plants and fungi, and they appear together with double strand breaks. Mutants deficient for spo11 show a failure of meiosis. However, induced breaks are regarded as part of a later evolution of meiosis [51]. The evolution of spo11 suggests that in early eukaryotes, the model of programmed double strand breaks generated by modern spo11 homologs is not applicable. In early protists, DSBs caused by oxidative damage might have been the direct trigger for spo11-like topoisomerase activity to cap the lesions which would prevent further lesions by ROS. Topoisomerases form tyrosyl phosphodiester links to the DNA backbone [52]. If the DNA backbone or the bases were already attacked and damaged by ROS before, then free oxygen radicals would hang around on loose ends either on the sugar-phosphate backbone or on the bases. Damaged DNA thus becomes a highly reactive radical by itself. In this situation, the electrons that are required to scavenge the radicals can be taken from the spo11 tyrosine, while a transesterase reaction links to the DNA backbone, thereby cleaving and sealing the end [53]. This action initiates the further steps of recombinational repair whereby spo11 remains initially attached to the cleaved ends and is later removed by endonucleases. Thus, spo11 may have a capping and marking function of oxidative damages, which initiates recombinational repair. According to this hypothesis, DSBs would not be *caused* by topoisomerase activity, but represent a consequence of topoisomerases reacting to DNA base oxidation, which marks the chromosome region requiring urgent repair. This is simply a chemical reaction following an oxidative damage, not a break on purpose. The enzyme machinery of meiosis then just needs to repair the DSB which confers an immediate selective advantage.

A repair function for DNA damages other than breaks can be inferred from the observations on *Tetrahymena* [45]. Thus, the main function of spo11 would be to seal ends and mark the damaged site before starting with repair. Other proteins, such as the MRN complex, then conduct single strand invasion, resulting in Holliday junctions and recombination during zygotene and early pachytene. These processes require all mitotic homologous repair components together with the meiosis-specific enzymes. Mismatch repair enzymes are normally important for eliminating replication errors to keep mutation rates down; MMR related enzymes act during meiosis for the resolution of Holliday junctions, or act in the rejection of crossing-over between divergent (non-homologous) chromosomes [46].

It is still unclear why spo11-induced cleavage is targeted to certain sites, so called "hot spots", while other regions are recombinationally rather stable [52]. In *Saccharomyces cerevisiae*, 150–300 DSBs are formed during prophase I prior to formation of the synaptonemal complex [54]; these DSBs are inducers of homologous recombination, and the lack of DSBs in mutants deficient for Spo11 blocks recombination. But, in fact, most of DSBs do NOT result in cross-overs. In plants, it is meanwhile established that around 90% of Holliday junctions are resolved as non-crossovers. That is, only 10% of spo11 induced DSBs would serve for efficient recombination. From this small percentage again only a part of new gene combinations in the flanking regions might be beneficial. Under the assumption that meiosis is good for creating new gene combinations, DSBs would resemble a lottery with perhaps 2-3% potential winners among the recombined products of meiosis. The recombined gametes further have to merge with gametes of another individual – without any guarantee that the new gene combination in the zygote would be favored by selection. That is, in the light of new findings on meiosis - recombination at meiosis becomes like a lottery where only few of the offspring would have the winners ticket, the great majority would have no benefit or even a disadvantage form an unfavorable new gene combination. From mathematical modelling, the lottery model for maintenance of sex [55] in general has been shown to be wrong as it would require a strong, truncating selection to give a benefit to a very small proportion of the offspring, that of the fittest, while the great majority of the offspring would have to be purged by selection. Since the assumption of truncating selection is an unrealistic assumption and the proportion of winners of meiotic recombination is far too small, the model was rejected as a general explanation for maintenance of sex.

A further paradox arises from a functional perspective: how should spo11 "know" whether the recombination at these sites would be beneficial? The "foresight" of evolution is already unrealistic for behavior of individuals, it is even more unrealistic for the activity of enzymes which simply follow the chemistry inherent in their molecular structures. So how could such an elaborate enzyme machinery evolve that would make a serious DNA lesion for the likelihood to win in a lottery? This lottery, is, as we know, a very expensive one, as a number of proteins have to be synthesized to conduct recombinational repair of an induced DSB. In fact, in the light of new findings on meiosis it seems that an additional cost has to be calculated, that of producing a big set of proteins for the whole meiosis machinery. From the perspective of a selective advantage, such a costly lottery ticket is unrealistic. It would be much more convincing to assume a direct and immediate benefit of DNA repair to meiotic products that can be immediately favored by selection. If DNA lesions are the trigger for the initiation of recombination then it is easier to explain that "hotspots" for recombination exist at sites where previous oxidative damage is severe; otherwise the observed topological distributions of recombination sites do not have any convincing functional explanation [50]. And, it is reasonable that in multicellular organisms, the costly and accurate homologous recombinational repair during meiosis I is focused on the germline cells, while other, less accurate and potentially mutagenic non-recombinational repair is good enough for somatic cells.

Meiosis is thus crucial for eukaryotic life. Even in asexual lineages, meiosis is hardly ever eliminated completely: in angiosperms, apomixis is usually facultative, i.e. sexual processes occur in parallel to apomictic reproduction, with low frequencies of meiotic offspring [56]. However, meiosis by itself has not been silenced, it takes place but is just by-passed by a somatic cell or altered to avoid the reduction of ploidy. Occasional sex, ie. normal meiosis and production of a reduced gametophyte, happens regularly at low frequenices. In animals, automixis is a widespread form of asexuality, but automixis maintains meiosis with meiotic products fused again [6]. Most strikingly, many forms of automixis result in homozygous offspring, with all its detrimental effects. To some extent automixis is more similar to self-fertilization of flowering plants (autogamy) which is usually regarded as a sexual process. In such cases, meiosis cannot be maintained because of recombination – it requires another function which is most likely DNA repair. That is, the key component of sex, the repair at meiosis I, is still present. Animals with cyclical parthenogenesis like Daphnias alternate between sexual and asexual generations, the former being produced under environmental stress situations [57]. All these forms of asexual or parasexual reproduction demonstrate that meiosis I has a crucial function other than creating new gene combinations.

5. The purging of deleterious mutations in diploid-haploid cycles

The DNA repair hypothesis explains the origin of programmed DSBs, the need for a second chromosome for recombinational repair, and the evolution of Holliday junctions. But, it does not explain the second important part of meiosis, ie. segregation of chromosomes at anaphase I, the lack of a second synthesis phase, and the subsequent mitotic division at meiosis II which results in four haploid meiotic products. For conducting recombinational repair, permanent diploidy would suffice [11]. This was one of the major points of criticism of the original repair hypothesis. The processes after prophase I cannot be related to DNA repair but must have another functional background. From a mechanical view, segregation could be a direct consequence of homolog pairing at prophase I, as synapsis and correct homolog pairing are required for correct segregation [51]. Wilkins and Holliday [51] discuss that the evolution of meiosis out of mitosis requires just a few alterations, basically the homolog pairing of chromosomes at prophase I, while the processes, i.e. skipping of centromere splitting and segregation of chromosomes instead of chromatids, and skipping the second S phase, are just consequences of homolog pairing. The authors discuss that these processes would have evolved to limit erroneous recombination. Although this hypothesis is convincing from a mechanical point of view it does not provide an evolutionary explanation of a selective advantage to maintain this as a regular process.

Here I will briefly summarize an idea proposed earlier by Hörandl [12] that reductional division is needed to eliminate mutations. Mutations, as changes in the DNA sequence, cannot be actively repaired; in fact they are mostly products of an erroneous non-homologous DNA repair mechanism [34]. Most mutations are either neutral or deleterious. Asexual lineages would accumulate deleterious mutations from generation to generation, while genotypes with low mutational load would be lost by drift in small populations; this process would in the long run lead to extinction of asexual lineages (Muller's ratchet; [15]). Recombination in a sexual population can reconstitute the genotypes with a lower load of mutations in the progeny, which was seen as a major advantage of sexuality. However, a lot of questions remain unanswered in this hypothesis. First, mutation accumulation happens far too slowly to give an immediate benefit to recombination; second, Muller's ratchet is only effective in small populations; third, the existence of ancient asexuals that had no sex for millions of years questions the generality of the model. Again, an evolutionary perspective helps to develop a causal model.

Early eukaryotes were probably haplontic, and so are algae, many fungi, and bryophytes. In haplonts and haplodiplonts, the diploid stage was just needed to conduct recombinational repair, but it was not the predominant stage for the normal cellular functions which were optimized for haploidy. Initially, segregation might have just evolved to return to the default haploidy, whereby skipping the second synthesis phase before the start of meiosis II could have evolved as a response to lack of nutrition or in a situation of starvation. Hunger was the trigger for meiotic cell divisions which is consistent with observations that e.g. yeasts start sporulation under starvation [58-59]. After mixis, two chromosome sets are available for repair during prophase I, but for continuing the cell cycle on the diploid level, resources were not sufficient, and the gene regulatory network was not yet adapted to work in the diploid condition. In this situation, a cell cycle mechanism without the need of a second synthesis phase, resulting in four haploid daughter cells, conferred a selective advantage over continuing a solely mitotic cell division on the diploid level. The shift between diploid and haploid stages was initially probably just a side effect of recombinational repair under oxidative stress and nutrient-poor conditions.

http://dx.doi.org/10.5772/56542

This side effect became important after a shift from haplontic to diplontic or diplohaplontic life cycles which occurred in metazoans and in vascular plants (ferns, lycophytes, and seed plants). A predominant diploid life cycle allows for the buffering of deleterious or disadvantageous mutations in somatic cells as a second homologue without this mutation is left [60-62]. The masking hypothesis states that diploidy will be favored over haploidy under free recombination because of masking deleterious recessive mutations, but is less likely to be favored when recombination rates are low [63]. Even if somatic deleterious mutations are not inherited, they decrease the fitness of a population. Masking confers an advantage to diploidy compared to haploidy in both sexual and asexual organisms [64]. Thus, masking increases temporarily the fitness of diploid or polyploid populations [62]. But, diploidy increases the mutational load. It was already recognized by Haldane in 1937 [65] that the mean fitness of a population depends more on the genome-wide deleterious mutation rate than on the effects of mutations. The equilibrium mean fitness of a population is reduced by approximately c U, where c is the ploidy level and U the mutation rate per haploid genome [66]. Under the conditions of equivalent mutation rates per base pair, the mutational load is thus higher in diploid than in haploid organisms. Under these conditions and in the absence of epistasis, haploids will have the lowest mutational load. The masking effect also reduces the efficiency of selection against such mutations as individuals carrying such masked mutations are not targeted by selection. Mutations can accumulate. But, in the haploid stage a deleterious mutation in a functional gene will be expressed and exposed to selection. If the mutational load strongly reduces the fitness of that individual, selection can purge the population from the mutations by eliminating the individual that carries the mutation. This way a haploid line can keep the mutational load low, especially if it has a rapid generation turnover, while a diploid line will accumulate mutations.

The diplontic or diplohaplontic organism would carry a lot of "masked" mutations after a prolonged diploid phase. After a return to the haploid phase, previously masked mutations are immediately exposed to selection which increases the efficiency of selection against mutants in the haploid gametes or gametophytes [12,49]. Segregation is quantitatively more important for the creation of new combinations of alleles than physical recombination [62]. Therefore, segregation at meiosis has a two-fold effect: creating genetic variation in the products of meiosis, and consequently among gametes or gametophytes, and expressing genes with deleterious mutations, which allows selection to act efficiently upon the fitness of haploid stages. This hypothesis would infer a strong selective advantage for a regular return to the haploid stage. In fact, selection on haploid gametes is always quite strong as few gametes, and only the fittest ones, reach syngamy and karyogamy; most of them are lost. In anisogamous organisms selection is usually very hard on male gametes, as spermatozoids usually must actively move and compete to win the race to the egg cell for fertilization. In flowering plants, competition is known even for the immobile male gametophyte: competition among pollen tubes occurs as they grow through the style and selects for the fastest ones [68]. It also makes sense that selection is usually weaker on the immobile female gametes, as their function is to keep cell organelles inactive to protect from oxidative stress [42]. Gametes or gametophytes of vascular plants are small, short-lived and thus can be produced in high numbers; it does not matter too much to lose the great majority of them in a hard truncating selection process which purges defective, non-competitive mutants as they have no chance to proceed to fertilization.

The mutations carried by these gametes or gametophytes are eliminated from the lineage, and the zygote can combine two "purged" chromosome sets. Thus, meiosis becomes a comprehensive DNA restoration process which eliminates not only direct defects of ROS but also indirect consequences, ie. mutations in germline cells.

The establishment of a reductional division requires mixis to re-establish the diploid stage. In all higher eukaryotes, such meiosis-mixis cycles become obligate from generation to generation as a regular DNA restoration process is essential for maintenance of a lineage [12].

6. Conclusions and directions for future research

Recent evidence strongly supports that meiosis not only originated for DNA restoration, but also that meiosis is maintained for this purpose in extant organisms. In addition to the benefits of DNA repair at prophase I the alteration of diploid-haploid cycles helps to purge mutations from the germline in diplontic or diplohaplontic organisms. Allelic recombination is just a by-product, a side effect of this process which does have other important evolutionary consequences, but is not the reason why sex is maintained [12].

The hypotheses proposed here are derived from observations of quite different research fields: redox chemistry, DNA function and repair, karyology and chromosome research, proteomics, eukaryotic bauplan (generalized body plan) and physiology, and evolutionary history. Further relevant information is needed in all these fields, but the challenge to combine results from different fields into a coherent theory is even greater. The main aim of this review is to stimulate broader interdisciplinary thinking, and to develop research projects to specifically test the different hypotheses of this theory.

Redox chemistry is a relatively young field, and it is still a challenge to reliably trace and measure reactions and results of oxidative damage on organic molecules. Most ROS are extremely unstable, with msec half times and thus difficult to measure in living tissues [69]. ROS may induce various different reactions not only with DNA and RNA molecules but also with other components of the cells. At low levels, ROS can be molecular messengers for many life-history traits [70], but at high levels they exert damaging effects. Most important, the role of oxidative stress and ROS on the onset and during meiosis, and the effects of ROS on meiosis protein-DNA interactions need further investigations.

DNA repair has become a major field of research and allowed for the recognition of the functional and evolutionary origin of meiosis out of DNA repair mechanisms. Nevertheless, the role of DNA repair during meiotic recombination in extant, modern eukaryotes is still not well understood. Most authors take it for granted that DSBs at meiosis are done "on purpose" but they disregard the chemical processes during the origin of DSBs. Recombination hotspots need to be investigated as to whether they represent damaged sites, as hypothesized here. Further studies on meiosis proteins and chromosome behavior under different levels of oxidative stress are needed to understand the postulated repair functions of meiosis.

http://dx.doi.org/10.5772/56542

Meiotic sex is ubiquitous in eukaryotes, but nevertheless many different physiological constraints and life forms exist in various eukaryotic groups. Most observations on sex as a response to oxidative stress have been made on organisms with a simple bauplan, such as algae, fission yeasts and protists. Detailed studies on the correlation of oxidative stress and sex in metazoans and land plants are still scarce. A major problem is the scarcity of suitable model systems with both sexual / asexual reproduction in higher eukaryotes to see effects of oxidative stress on mode of reproduction. In animals, abiotic stress affects the reproduction mode in animals with cyclic parthenogenesis, e.g. daphnias and aphids [57]. However, for mammals as the best established lab organisms, no natural parthenogenesis is known. The germline of metazoans separates very early in development, and is thus kept apart from the tissues with the highest oxidative stress (e.g., muscles, liver cells). It will be crucial to investigate stress responses and putative signalling or messenger pathways between germline and somatic cells, and different constraints on male and female gamete formation. In plants, environmental stress leads to increased frequencies of homologous recombination, both in meiosis and mitosis, and epigenetic instability [71]. Plants have the advantage that germline cells (megaspore and microspore mother cells) differentiate late in the development in adult individuals; thus, meiosis can potentially be directly correlated to environmental stress factors, which makes them suitable for experimental approaches. Nevertheless, few model systems allow for a comparison of sexual and asexual reproduction. Transcriptomic studies on sexual / asexual *Boechera* show a significant increase of oxidoreductase gene activity during the promeiotic to the meiotic stage. Genes that were overall significantly over-represented in meiotic stages in sexual plants compared to apomictic plants include those related to redox regulation [72-73]. It will be promising to study oxidative stress, gene expression, and mode of reproduction in facultatively apomictic flowering plants under different environmental stress conditions.

The hypothesis on purging mutations in haploid stages can only be tested on diplontic or diplohaplontic organisms, i.e. animals or seed plants. Ferns are also theoretically interesting, but high ploidy levels might complicate methodological setups. It might be promising to study model organisms forming unreduced gamete and gametophytes, and their offspring with respect to mutational load compared to the parental organisms. Unreduced gametes are expected to result in offspring with a higher mutational load than in model systems with reduced gametes / gametophytes as the purging effect should be weakened. Genomic approaches will be needed to detect changes among generations. Moreover, it will be important to study gene expression in gametes / gametophytes to understand genes that set the fitness parameters on which selection can act upon during the insemination / pollination and fertilization process. Finally, mathematical modeling is promising for understanding long term effects of gamete selection over many generations, as diplontic organisms mostly have a slow generation turnover.

Acknowledgements

I would like to thank John Carman and Ingo Schubert for general discussions on sex, and Franz Hadacek for valuable comments on the manuscript concerning redox chemistry. Financial support from the Austrian Science Fund (FWF; Project I 310-B03) and from the German Science Fund (DFG project Ho-4395) is gratefully acknowledged.

Author details

Elvira Hörandl*

Address all correspondence to: elvira.hoerandl@biologie.uni-goettingen.de

Dept. Systematic Botany, Albrecht-von-Haller Institute for Plant Sciences, University of Göttingen, Göttingen, Germany

References

[1] Otto S. The evolutionary enigma of sex. Amer Nat. 2009;171 (Suppl.): 1-14.

[2] Lewis WM jr. The cost of sex. In: Stearns SC. (ed.) The evolution of sex and its consequences, Basel: Birkhäuser; 1987. p33—57.

[3] Maynard Smith J. The Evolution of Sex. Cambridge: Cambridge University Press; 1978.

[4] Bell G. The Masterpiece of Nature: the Evolution and Genetics of Sexuality. California Press: Berkeley; 1982.

[5] Burt A. Perspective: Sex, recombination and the efficacy of selection-was Weismann right? Evolution 2000;54(2): 337—351.

[6] Engelstädter J. Constraints on the evolution of asexual reproduction. Bioessays 2008;30(11): 1138-1150.

[7] Koltunow A, Grossniklaus U. Apomixis, a developmental perspective. Annual Review of Plant Biology 2003; 54: 547—574.

[8] Hörandl E, Hojsgaard D. The evolution of apomixis in angiosperms – a reappraisal. Plant Biosystems 2012;146(3): 681-693.

[9] Cavalier-Smith T. Origin of the cell nucleus, mitosis and sex: roles of intracellular coevolution. Biology Direct 2010;5: 7.

[10] Mogie, M, Britton NF, Stewart-Cox, JA. Asexuality, polyploidy and the male function. In: Hörandl E, Grossniklaus U, Sharbel T, van Dijk P (eds.) Apomixis: Evolution, Mechanisms and Perspectives. Gantner Verlag: Ruggell; 2007. p195-214.

[11] Birdsell JA, Wills C. The evolutionary origin and maintenance of sexual recombination: a review of contemporary models. Evolutionary Biology 2003;33: 27—138.

[12] Hörandl E. A combinational theory for maintenance of sex. Heredity 2009;103(6): 445–457.

[13] Fisher RA. The Genetical Theory of Natural Selection. Clarendon Press, Oxford; 1930.

[14] Van Valen L. A new evolutionary law. Evolutionary Theory 1973;1(1): 1-30.

[15] Muller HJ. The relation of recombination to mutational advance. Mutation Research 1964;1: 2-9.

[16] Kondrashov AS. Deleterious mutations and the evolution of sexual reproduction. Nature 1988;336(6198): 435-440.

[17] Brooks LA. The evolution of recombination rates. In: Michod RE, Levin BR (eds.) The Evolution of Sex, Massachusetts: Sinauer Ass.;1988. p. 87—105.

[18] Bernstein, H, Byerly, H, Hopf, F, Michod RE. Is meiotic recombination an adaptation for repairing DNA, producing genetic variation, or both? In: Michod RE, Levin BR (eds.) The Evolution of Sex, Massachusetts: Sinauer Ass.;1988. p139—160.

[19] Bernstein C, Bernstein H. Aging, Sex and DNA repair. San Diego: Academic Press, 1991.

[20] Bernstein C. Sex as a response to oxidative damage. In: Halliwell B, Aruoma OI (eds.) DNA & Free Radicals. Techniques, mechanisms, & applications. OICA international. London: Saint Lucia; 1998. p99-118.

[21] Margulis L, Sagan D. Origins of Sex: Three Billion Years of Genetic Recombination. New Haven: Yale University Press. 1986.

[22] Halliwell B. Reactive species and antioxidants. Redox biology is a fundamental theme of aerobic life. Plant Physiology 2006;141(2): 312-322.

[23] Cohen Y, Jorgensen BB, Revsbech NP, Poplawski R. Adaptation to Hydrogen Sulfide of oxygenic and anoxygenic photosynthesis among Cyanobacteria. Applied and Environmental Microbiology, 1986(2): 398-407.

[24] Allen JF. A redox switch hypothesis for the origin of two light reactions in photosynthesis. FEBS Letters 2005;579(5): 963–968.

[25] Blankenship RE, Hartman H. The origin and evolution of oxygenic photosynthesis. Trends in Biochemical Sciences 1998;23(3): 94-97.

[26] Kasting JF. Earth history – the rise of atmospheric oxygen. Science 2001;293(5531): 819-820.

[27] Catlin DC, Glein CR, Zahnle KJ, McKay CP. Why O_2 Is required by complex life on habitable planets and the concept of planetary "Oxygenation Time". Astrobiology 2005;5(3): 415-438.

[28] Rinalducci S, Murgiano L, Zolla L. Redox proteomics: basic principles and future perspectives for the detection of protein oxidation in plants. Journal of Experimental Botany 2008;59(14): 3781–3801.

[29] Roldan-Arjona T., Ariza RR. Repair and tolerance of oxidative DNA damage in plants. Mutation Research 2009;681(2-3): 169–179.

[30] Martin W, Müller M. The hydrogen hypothesis for the first eukaryote. Nature 1998;392(6671): 37-41.

[31] Kowaltowski AJ, de Souza-Pinto NC, Castilho RF, Vercesi AE. Mitochondria and reactive oxygen species. Free Radical Biology & Medicine 2009;47(4): 333–343.

[32] Epe B. DNA damage induced by photosynthesizers and photoreactive compounds. In: Aruoma OI, Halliwell B. (eds.) DNA and free radicals. Techniques, Mechanisms and Applications. Saint Lucia, London: OICA international; 1998;p 63--96.

[33] Dizdaroglu M. Mechanisms of free radical damage to DNA. In: Aruoma OI, Halliwell B. (eds.) DNA and free radicals. Techniques, Mechanisms and Applications. Saint Lucia, London: OICA international; 1998;p3--26.

[34] Friedberg EC, Walker GC, Siede W, Wood, RD, Schultz, RA, Ellenberger T. DNA Repair and Mutagenesis. 2n ed. Washington D.C.: American Society for Microbiology; 2006.

[35] Bergeron F, Auvre F, Radicella JP, Ravanat, JL. HO• radicals induce an unexpected high proportion of tandem base lesions refractory to repair by DNA glycosylases. Proceedings of the National Academy of Sciences of the United States of America 2010;107(12): 5528-5533.

[36] Pfannschmidt T, Bräutigam K, Wagner R, Dietzel L, Schröter Y, Steiner S, Nykytenko A. Potential regulation of gene expression in photosynthetic cells by redox and energy state: approaches towards better understanding. Annals of Botany 2009;103(4): 599–607.

[37] Apel K, Hirt H. Reactive oxygen species: Metabolism, oxidative stress, and signal transduction. Annu. Rev. Plant Biology 2004;55: 373-399.

[38] Bleuyard, J-Y, Gallego, ME, White, CI Recent advances in understanding of the DNA double-strand break repair machinery of plants. DNA repair 2006;5(1): 1-12.

[39] Li X, Heyer, WD. Homologous recombination in DNA repair and DNA damage tolerance. Cell Research 2008;18(1): 99-113

[40] Svendsen JM, Harper JW. GEN1/Yen1 and the SLX4 complex: solutions to the problem of Holliday junction resolution. Genes and Development 2010; 24(6): 521-536.

[41] Jackson SP, Bartek J. The DNA-damage response in human biology and disease. Nature 2009;461(7267): 1071-1078.

[42] Allen JF Separate sexes and the mitochondrial theory of ageing. Journal of Theoretical Biology 1996;180(2): 135-140.

[43] Nedelcu AM, Michod RE. Sex as a response to oxidative stress: the effect of antioxidants on sexual induction in a facultatively sexual lineage. Proceedings of the Royal Society of London B 2003;270(Suppl.): S136-S139.

[44] Nedelcu AM. Marco O, Michod RE. Sex as a response to oxidative stress: a twofold increase in cellular reactive oxygen species activates sex genes. Proc. R. Soc. Lond. B 2004;271(1548): 1591-1596

[45] Loidl J, Mochizuki K. Tetrahymena meiotic nuclear reorganization is induced by a checkpoint Kinase–dependent response to DNA damage. Molecular Biology of the Cell 2009;20(9): 2428–2437

[46] Egel R, Penny L. On the origin of meiosis in eukaryotic evolution: coevolution of meiosis and mitosis from feeble beginnings. In: Lankenau, DH Egel R (eds). Sex and Recombination: Models, Means and Evolution. Berlin: Springer;2007.p249-288.

[47] Ramesh MA, Malik SB, Logsdon JM. A phylogenomic inventory of meiotic genes: evidence for sex in Giardia and an early eukaryotic origin of meiosis. Current Biology 2005;15(2): 185–191.

[48] Malik, SB, Ramesh MA, Hulstrand AM, Logsdon JM. Protist homologs of the meiotic Spo11 gene and Topoisomerase VI reveal an evolutionary history of gene duplication and lineage-specific loss. Molecular Biology Evolution 2007; 24(12): 2827–2841

[49] Schubert, I. 2011. 'Sex and crime' in evolution - why sexuality was so successful. Genes & Genetic Systems 86(1): 1-6.

[50] Schurko AM, Logsdon JM. Using a meiosis detection toolkit to investigate ancient asexual "scandals" and the evolution of sex. BioEssays 2008;30(6): 579-589.

[51] Wilkins AS, Holliday R. The evolution of meiosis from mitosis. Genetics 2009;181(1): 3-12.

[52] Keeney S. Spo11 and the formation of DNA Double-Strand Breaks in meiosis. In: Egel R, Lankenau, DH (eds.) Recombination and Meiosis. Crossing over and Disjunction. Berlin: Springer; 2010. p81-124.

[53] Hörandl E, Hadacek F. submitted. The oxidative damage initiation hypothesis for meiosis. Plant Reproduction.

[54] Richardson C, Horikoshi, N, Pandita TK. The role of the DNA double-strand break response network in meiosis. DNA Repair 2004;3(8-9): 1149–1164.

[55] Williams GS. Sex and Evolution. Princeton: Princeton University Press; 1975.

[56] Hörandl E, Paun O. Patterns and sources of genetic diversity in apomictic plants: implications for evolutionary potentials. In: Hörandl E., Grossniklaus U., van Dijk P.,

Sharbel, T. (eds.), Apomixis: Evolution, Mechanisms and Perspectives, 2007. p169-194. Gantner Verlag: Ruggell, Liechtenstein.

[57] Suomolainen E, Saura A, Lokki J. Cytology and Evolution of Parthenogenesis. Boca Raton: CRC Press;1987.

[58] Margulis L, Sagan D. Origins of Sex: Three Billion Years of Genetic Recombination. New Haven: Yale University Press;1986.

[59] Cavalier-Smith T. The phagotrophic origin of eukaryotes and phylogenetic classification of protozoa. International Journal of Systematic and Evolutionary Microbiology 2002;52: 297-354.

[60] Crow JF, Kimura M. An Introduction to Population Genetics Theory., New York: Harper and Row;1970.

[61] Kondrashov AS, Crow JF. Haploidy or diploidy: which is better? Nature 1991;351(6324): 314 – 315.

[62] Otto SP, Whitton J. Polyploidy incidence and evolution. Annual Review of Genetics 2000;34: 401-437.

[63] Otto SP, Goldstein DB. Recombination and the evolution of diploidy. Genetics 1992;131(3): 745—751.

[64] Orr HA. Somatic mutation favors the evolution of diploidy. Genetics 1995;139(3): 1441-1447.

[65] Haldane JBS. The effect of variation on fitness. American Naturalist 1937;71:337-349.

[66] Gerstein AC, Otto SP. Ploidy and causes of genomic evolution. Journal of Heredity 2009;100(5): 571-581.

[67] Crow JF. The importance of recombination. In: Michod RE, Levin BR (eds.) The Evolution of Sex. Massachusetts: Sinauer Ass.; 1988. p56—73.

[68] Erbar C. Pollen-tube transmitting tissue: place of competition of male gametophytes. International Journal of Plant Sciences 2003;164(Suppl.): S265-S277.

[69] Bonini MG, Rota, C, Tomasi A, Mason RP. The oxidation of 2 ',7 '-dichlorofluorescin to reactive oxygen species: A self-fulfilling prophesy? Free Radical Biology and Medicine 2006;40(6): 968-975.

[70] Dowling DK, Simmons, LW. Reactive oxygen species as universal constraints in life history evolution. Proceedings of the Royal Society B. 2009;276(1663): 1737-1745.

[71] Boyko A, Kovalchuk I. Genome instability and epigenetic modification - heritable responses to environmental stress? Current Opinion in Plant Biology 2011;14(3): 260-266.

[72] Sharbel TF, Voigt ML, Corral JM, Thiel T, Varshney A, Kuhmlehn J, Vogel H, Rotter, B. Molecular signatures of apomictic and sexual ovules in the Boechera holboellii complex. Plant Journal 2009;58(5): 870–882.

[73] Sharbel TF, Voigt ML, Corral JM, Galla G, Kuhmlehn J, Klukas C, Schreiber F, Vogel H, Rotter B. Apomictic and sexual ovules of Boechera display heterochronic global gene expression patterns. Plant Cell 2010;22(3): 655–671.

Chapter 3

Evolutionary Origin and Adaptive Function of Meiosis

Harris Bernstein and Carol Bernstein

Additional information is available at the end of the chapter

http://dx.doi.org/10.5772/56557

1. Introduction

The origin of meiosis and its adaptive function in eukaryotes, and the related problem of the origin and adaptive function of sex in eukaryotes, are fundamental issues in biology. Among eukaryotes, meiosis and sexual reproduction are widespread, occurring in single-celled eukaryotes (including protozoans such as paramecium), and fungi (e.g. yeast) and in most multicellular organisms including animals and most plants. Accumulating evidence indicates that meiosis arose very early in the evolution of eukaryotes (reviewed in Bernstein & Bernstein, 2010). Thus, basic features of meiosis were likely already present in the prokaryotic ancestors of eukaryotes.

Central features of meiosis are the pairing of homologous chromosomes of different parental origin, recombination (information exchange) between these chromosomes, and the passage of the recombined chromosomes to progeny. In bacteria, the sexual process of transformation has these same essential features (Michod et al., 2008). In a further parallel, key enzymes that catalyze meiotic recombination are homologous to enzymes that serve similar functions in the recombinational steps of transformation. The earliest eukaryotic organisms were single-celled protists, similar to bacteria. In this chapter we review the evidence that meiosis in the earliest single-celled eukaryotes evolved from the sexual process of transformation in their bacterial ancestors.

Among extant organisms, both single-celled bacteria and single-celled eukaryotes tend to enter the sexual cycle under conditions of environmental stress (Bernstein & Bernstein, 2010). These are conditions that can cause DNA damage. DNA damage appears to be an important fundamental problem for all organisms. We review evidence here that DNA damaging agents induce sex in prokaryotes and microbial eukaryotes. We summarize evidence in bacterial transformation and in eukaryotic meiosis that recombination serves the adaptive function of removing DNA damages that are potentially lethal to progeny (see also Bernstein & Bernstein, 2004; Bernstein et al., 2011).

Thus in this chapter we explore the reasoned likelihood that meiotic recombination arose from bacterial transformation and that both transformation and meiosis are adaptations for repairing damage in the DNA to be passed on to progeny.

2. The common ancestor of all eukaryotes was likely capable of meiosis

Eukaryotes emerged from prokaryotic ancestors more than 1.5 billion years ago (Javaux et al., 2001). The oldest taxonomically resolved eukaryote in the fossil record, *Bangiomorph pubescens*, a red algae, existed more than 1.2 billion years ago and was sexually reproducing (Butterfield, 2000). Although meiotic sex is widespread among extant eukaryotes, it has, until recently, been unclear whether or not eukaryotes were sexual early in their evolution. The reason for this uncertainty was that sexual reproduction and meiosis appeared to be absent in certain eukaryotes thought to belong to lineages that diverged early in eukaryote evolution. However, due to recent advances in gene detection and other techniques, an increasing number of the presumed "ancient asexual" eukaryotes are now known to be capable of, or to recently have had the capacity, to undergo meiosis and hence sexual reproduction.

Thus, the common intestinal parasite *Giardia intestinalis* was once thought to be an asexual descendant of a eukaryotic lineage that arose prior to the emergence of meiosis and sex, but it was recently found to have a core set of meiotic genes, including five genes known to be specific to meiosis (Ramash et al., 2005). Evidence indicative of current sexual reproduction in present day *Giardia intestinalis* has now also been found (Cooper et al., 2007). In another example, a sexual cycle was recently found in parasitic protozoa of the genus *Leishmania* (Akopyants et al., 2009).

Trichomonas vaginalis is a unicellular parasitic eukaryote. Although not known to currently undergo meiosis, this capability was likely present in a recent ancestor of this organism. This conclusion is based on the work of Malik et al. (2008) who tested *Trichomonas vaginalis* for the presence of 29 genes involved in meiosis and found 27 of these meiosis genes to be present, including 8 of 9 genes specific to meiosis in model organisms. Of the 27 meiotic genes that were present in *Trichomonas vaginalis*, 21 were also present in *Giardia intestinalis*. This finding indicates that most of the meiotic genes were present in a common ancestor of these two species. Since these species are descendants of separate lineages that diverged very early in the evolution of eukaryotes, Malik et al. (2008) suggested that each of the genes held in common was present in the common ancestor of all eukaryotes. Dacks and Roger (1999) also proposed, on the basis of a phylogenetic analysis, that facultative sex was present in the common ancestor of all eukaryotes. Lahr et al. (2011) recently reported evidence from a study of amoebae that supports this view. Even though amoebae are conventionally considered to be asexual, these authors presented evidence that most amoeboid lineages were at one time sexual, and that most asexual groups probably arose recently and independently.

Another group of eukaryotes, commonly referred to as a member of the "ancient asexuals," the arbuscular mycorrhizal fungi, were thought to have propagated colonally for over 500 million years. However, recently, several members of this group (*Glomus spp.*) were shown to possess in their genome homologs of 51 meiotic genes including seven meiosis-specific genes, suggesting that their meiotic machinery has been conserved (Halary et al., 2011). The pathogenic yeast *Candida albicans* had been long regarded as an "asexual" eukaryote. However, it is now known that this organism has maintained an elaborate—but largely hidden—mating apparatus (Johnson, 2003).

Thus, the common ancestor of current day eukaryotes was likely capable of meiosis.

3. Natural bacterial transformation as a form of sex

Natural bacterial transformation involves the transfer of DNA from one bacterium to another through the surrounding medium. Transformation depends on the expression of numerous bacterial genes whose products appear to be designed to carry out this process (Chen and Dubnau, 2004; Johnsborg et al., 2007). Transformation is ordinarily a complex, energy requiring developmental process. In order for a bacterium to bind, take up and recombine exogenous DNA into its chromosome it must enter a special physiological state, referred to as competence. Development of competence in *Bacillus subtilis* requires expression of about 40 genes (Solomon and Grossman, 1996). The exogenous DNA integrated into the recipient chromosome is usually (with rare exceptions) derived from another bacterium of the same species, and is thus homologous to the resident chromosome. The amount of DNA transferred during transformation can be a large portion, or the full length, of the bacterial chromosome (Akamatsu and Taguchi, 2001; Saito et al., 2006). The capacity for natural transformation appears to be common in nature, and thus far 67 prokaryotic species (in seven different phyla) are known to undergo this process (Johnsborg et al., 2007). As understanding of the behavior of other bacterial species under crowded conditions, such as in biofilms, continues to advance, many further examples of transformation are likely to be discovered. Transformation in bacteria can be viewed as a primitive sexual process, since it involves interaction of homologous DNA from two individuals to form recombinant DNA that is passed on to succeeding generations.

Transformation is similar to eukaryotic sex involving hydrophilus pollination in plants, in which water is a vector in the transportation of pollen (Cox, 1988). In both bacterial transformation and sex in such plants, DNA is passed from one individual to another through the intervening liquid medium, rather than by direct contact. On the other hand, an intermediate stage in the evolution of prokaryotic to eukaryotic sex may have been similar to sexual interaction in the extant archaebacterium *Halobacterium volcanii* that involves direct contact, similar to sexual interaction in paramecium and yeast. *Halobacterium volcanii* have a distinctive mating system in which cytoplasmic bridges between cells appear to be used for transfer of DNA from one cell to another in either direction (Rosenshine et al., 1989). In another similar bacterial system involving direct contact, Frols et al. (2008) showed that exposure of the archaebacterium *Sulfolobus solfataricus* to the DNA damaging agents UV-irradiation, bleomycin or mitomycin C induced cellular aggregation. Aggregation was not inducible by other physical stressors, such as pH or temperature shift, suggesting that induction is caused specifically by DNA damage. Frols et al. (2008; 2009) hypothesized that cellular aggregation enhances DNA transfer among *Sulfolobus* cells to provide increased repair of damaged DNA via homologous recombination. In related work, Wood et al. (1997) found that UV-irradiation of the thermophilic archaebacterium *Sulfolobus acidocaldarius* increased the frequency of recombination due to genetic exchange.

The transformation systems and archaebacterial systems appear to differ fundamentally from the more well-studied *E. coli* conjugation that is mediated by a parasitic plasmid (F-factor). In the bacterial transformation systems and archaebacterial systems, the genes promoting the sexual process of DNA transfer are presumably encoded in the bacterial genome, while for conjugation in *E. coli*, the genes governing conjugation are encoded in the parasitic plasmid.

4. Transformation and meiosis are similar at a molecular level

Bacterial transformation and eukaryotic meiosis are similar in their central molecular processes, and these processes are catalyzed by homologous gene products. There are three major steps in bacterial transformation: (1) DNA derived from a donor cell enters into a recipient cell; (2) the two homologous chromosomes (or homologous portions of the two chromosomes) derived from the two bacterial cells align and undergo genetic recombination (exchange of genetic information); (3) the new recombined chromosome is passed on to progeny bacteria. Meiosis in diploid eukaryotic cells can similarly be viewed as occurring by three steps. These steps are: (1) gametes undergo syngamy/fertilization so that chromosomes of different cellular origin share the same nucleus; (2) homologous chromosomes from different cells (i.e. non-sister chromosomes) align in pairs and undergo recombination; (3) two successive cell divisions (without chromosome duplication) lead to haploid gametes, which can repeat the cycle in subsequent generations. In meiosis, as in transformation, the central step (step 2) is the intimate alignment of non-sister homologous chromosomes followed by genetic recombination. In bacteria, recombination between non-sister homologous chromosomes is catalyzed by the RecA protein, and in eukaryotes this same reaction is catalyzed by orthologs of RecA, such as Rad51 and Dmc1 (see section 16, below).

5. The prokaryotic ancestor of eukaryotes was likely capable of transformation

The hypothesis that meiosis evolved from transformation depends on the assumption that the prokaryotic ancestor of the eukaryotic cell lineage was able to undergo transformation. A crucial event in the emergence of the eukaryotic cell was likely the establishment of a stable association of an anaerobic host bacterium and a smaller, internalized aerobic bacterium. We next consider the likelihood that this progenitor of the eukaryotic cell lineage was capable of transformation. The internalized aerobic bacterium is assumed to have provided the capacity for respiration, and to have eventually evolved into the mitochondrion. We will first focus on the nature of the internalized aerobe, and then on its anaerobic host.

On the basis of genome sequence analysis, extant mitochondria are most closely related to α-proteobacteria, suggesting that mitochondria are descended from an α-proteobacterium (Gray et al., 1999; Muller and Martin, 1999). Based on a computational analysis, Boussau et al. (2004) concluded that the common ancestor of α-proteobacteria likely had a genome consisting of between 3000 and 5000 genes, and was an aerobic, motile bacterium with pili and surface proteins for interacting with host cells. A gene sequence data analysis by Gray et al. (1999) strongly indicated a monophyletic origin of mitochondria from an α-proteobacterial ancestor, and also implied that mitochondria evolved only once. We can assess the plausibility of the idea that such an ancestor was capable of transformation by knowing whether present day α-proteobacteria are capable of transformation. In fact, several present day α-proteobacteria are capable of natural transformation, including *Agrobacterium tumefaciens* (Demaneche et al., 2001), *Methylobacterium organophilum* (O'Connor et al., 1977) and *Bradyrhizobium japonicum* (Raina and Modi, 1972).

The ancient anaerobic bacterial host of the internalized proto-mitochondrion was determined on the basis of a phylogenetic analysis to likely be an archaebacterium (Cox et al., 2008). Transformation has been reported among currently living archaebacteria including *Methanococcus voltae* (Bertani and Baresi, 1987; Patel et al., 1994), *Methanobacterium thermaautotrophicum* (Worrell et al., 1988) and *Halobacterium volcani* (Cline et al., 1989). On the basis of the known transformation capabilities of extant bacteria, it is a reasonable possibility that when the eukaryotic lineage first emerged, presumably by the association of an archaebacterium and an α-proteobacterium, at least one and possibly both of the partners were capable of transformation.

Evidence indicates that, during the evolution of mitochondria from an ancestral α-proteobacterium, much of the genetic information of the α-proteobacterium was transferred to, and became integrated into, the host nuclear genome. Phylogenetic studies by Gabaldon and Huynen (2003) suggest that at least 630 genes were transferred to the nuclear genome from the α-proteobacterial genome. If the ancestral α-proteobacterium was capable of transformation, as are some of its current day relatives, its genes necessary for transformation may have been integrated into the early eukaryotic nuclear genome. In current-day organisms, the gene family *RecA/Rad51/Dmc1* is central to the machinery of both bacterial transformation and meiotic recombination. The *RecA* orthologs in eukaryotes have a high level of sequence similarity to *RecA* genes from proteobacteria. Lin et al. (2006) suggested that transfer of the *RecA* gene from the early pre-mitochondria to the nuclear genome of ancestral eukaryotes could be the cause of this sequence similarity. Alternatively, *recA*-like genes from the archaebacterial ancestor may have given rise to the *rad51/dmc1* genes of eukaryotes as suggested by the work of Sandler et al. (1996). Thus genes central to eukaryotic meiosis could have been derived from genes central to transformation in a prokaryote. In subsequent sections we will argue that the adaptive function of transformation in the early prokaryotic predecessors of eukaryotes and of meiosis in their eukaryotic descendents is repair of DNA damage. However, first we discuss evidence that DNA damage is an important fundamental difficulty with which life must cope.

6. DNA damage is a basic problem for life

A DNA damage is an alteration in the molecular structure of DNA, such as a break in one or both DNA strands, a missing base, or an oxidized base (e.g. 8-OHdG). Damage to DNA often results from natural processes. As noted by Haynes (1988), DNA is comprised of rather ordinary molecular subunits that are not endowed with any unusual quantum mechanical stability, and this "chemical vulgarity" makes DNA vulnerable to all the "chemical horrors" that might befall any such molecule in a warm aqueous environment. The particular types of DNA damage occurring when organisms were undergoing the prokaryotic to eucaryotic transition cannot be determined directly, but can be indirectly surmised from the types of DNA damage occurring in present day organisms. In extant cellular organisms, metabolism releases numerous compounds that damage DNA including reactive oxygen species, reactive nitrogen species, reactive carbonyl species, lipid peroxidation products and alkylating compounds, among others, while hydrolysis cleaves chemical bonds in DNA (De Bont and van Larebeke, 2004). In eukaryotes such as mammals, tens to hundreds of thousands of naturally caused DNA damages occur per cell per day (see next section). While most of these DNA damages can be repaired, such repair is not 100% efficient. Unrepaired DNA damages accumulate, especially in non-replicating or slowly replicating cells.

One indication that DNA damages are a major problem for life is that DNA repair processes, to cope with ubiquitously occurring DNA damages, have been found in all cellular organisms in which DNA repair has been investigated. For example, in bacteria, a regulatory network aimed at repairing DNA damages (called the SOS response in *Escherichia coli*) has been found in many bacterial species. *E. coli* RecA, a key enzyme in the SOS response pathway, is the defining member of a ubiquitous class of DNA strand-exchange proteins that are essential for homologous recombinational repair, a pathway that maintains genomic integrity by repairing broken DNA (Bell et al., 2012). Eukaryotic recombinases that are homologues of RecA are also widespread in eukaryotes. For example, in fission yeast and humans, RecA homologues promote duplex-duplex DNA-strand exchange needed for repair of many types of DNA damages (Murayama et al., 2008; Holthausen et al., 2010).

Another indication that DNA damages are a major problem for life is that cells make large investments in DNA repair processes. As pointed out by Hoeijmakers (2009), repairing just one double-strand break may require more than 10,000 ATP molecules, since ATP is used in signaling the presence of the damage, the generation of repair foci, and the formation (in humans) of nucleofilament intermediates in homologous recombinational repair by RAD51, a homologue of bacterial RecA.

In plants, dormant seeds accumulate DNA damages which can be largely repaired during germination (Cheah and Osborne, 1978; Koppen and Verschaeve, 2001). Multiple effective

http://dx.doi.org/10.5772/56557

pathways for DNA damage signalling and repair have evolved in plants for dealing with endogenous and exogenous sources of DNA damage (reviewed by Bray and West, 2005).

Sagan (1973) examined the flux of solar UV irradiation penetrating the primitive reducing atmosphere of earth prior to the formation of a shielding ozone layer, and concluded that a mean lethal dose would be delivered to unprotected microorganisms of the type existing today in 0.3 seconds or less. Since DNA damage is the main cause of UV-induced lethality, it appears that DNA damage was likely a problem for even the earliest microorganisms.

7. Frequency of occurrence and consequences of DNA damage

An idea of the magnitude of the biologic problem posed by naturally occuring DNA damage can be obtained by considering the frequency of occurrence and consequences of DNA damages in present day organisms. The estimated frequency of occurrence of oxidative DNA damages per cell per day is about 10,000 in humans (Ames et al., 1993; Helbock et al., 1998) and about 74,000 to 100,000 in rats (Fraga et al., 1990; Ames et al., 1993; Helbock et al., 1998). For depurinations, the estimated frequency is 9,000 to 13,920, per mammalian cell per day (Nakamura et al., 1998; Tice and Setlow, 1985); for single-strand breaks, the frequency is about 55,200 per cell per day (Tice and Setlow, 1985). Double-strand breaks, which are difficult to repair accurately, occur in human cells at a frequency estimated to be 10 (Haber, 1999) to 50 (Vilenchik & Knudson, 2003) per cell cycle. Other types of DNA damage, such as formation of O^6-methylguanine and cytosine deamination are also frequent.

An unrepaired DNA damage may block replication of the DNA, and when such a damage occurs in the transcribed strand, it may also block RNA polymerase catalysed transcription (Kathe et al., 2004). Blockage of DNA replication can be lethal to a cell, and blockage of transcription is deleterious because it can interfere with the synthesis of a protein coded for by the gene in which a blockage occurs.

Also, during DNA replication, as the DNA polymerase copies a DNA strand containing a damaged site, it may inaccurately bypass the damage and in so doing generate a mutation. Although damages and mutations are both errors in DNA, DNA damages are distinct from mutations. DNA damages are structural and chemical alterations in the DNA, whereas mutations ordinarily involve the normal four bases in new arrangements. Furthemore, whereas DNA damages are altered structures that cannot be replicated, mutations can be replicated when the DNA replicates. In aerobically growing bacteria, reactive oxygen species (ROS) seem to be an important source of DNA damage, as indicated by the observation that 89% of spontaneously occurring base substitution mutations are caused by inaccurate replication past bases damaged by ROS (Sakai et al., 2006). Thus another harmful consequence of DNA damages is that they likely generate a substantial portion of spontaneous mutations.

Further consequences of DNA damages for eukaryotes and prokaryotes are the expenditures of energy, time and material resoures (e.g. nucleotides) required by the multiple processes that repair DNA damages. Five major pathways are employed in repairing various kinds of DNA damages. These processes are nucleotide excision repair, base excision repair, mismatch repair, non-homologous end joining and homologous recombinational repair (HRR) [reviewed in Bernstein et al. (2002)]. Only one of the five pathways, HRR, is able to accurately repair double-strand damages, such as double-strand breaks (DSBs). The HRR pathway depends on the availability of second homologous chromosome for restoring the information lost by the first chromosome due to the DSB. As detailed below, in both prokaryotes and eukaryotes, sex promotes the conditions needed for especially effective HRR of double-strand damages.

Overall, it is clear that, in eukaryotes and prokaryotes, DNA damages are ubiquitous and thus are a major problem for cellular and organismal survival. Furthermore, over time, DNA damages have selected for the evolution of numerous complex, specialized DNA repair pathways.

8. Competence for transformation is induced by stress in prokaryotes

Both transformation and meiosis (in microbial eukaryotes) are induced by stressful conditions. Thus transformation may have evolved by natural selection as an adaptive response to stress in prokaryotes and been maintained for this purpose subsequent to the transition to meiotic sex. In this section we describe stressful conditions that induce competence for transformation and in section 10 we describe similar stressful conditions that induce meiotic sex in eukaryotic microorganisms.

Among present day bacteria, competence for transformation is induced when bacteria are grown to high cell density and/or under nutritional limitation, conditions characteristic of the stationary phase of bacterial growth. As an example, transformation in *Haemophilus influenzae* occurs most efficiently at the end of exponential growth as cells approach stationary phase (Goodgal and Herriott, 1961). In *Streptococcus mutans,* as well as many other streptococci, transformation occurs at high cell density, especially during biofilm formation (Aspiras et al., 2004). Competence in *Bacillus subtilis* is induced toward the end of logarithmic growth, particularly under conditions of amino acid limitation (Anagnostopoulos and Spizizen, 1961). Michod et al. (2008) reviewed evidence suggesting that, in the inflammatory oxidizing environment associated with infection, transformation in pathogenic bacteria (i.e. *Neisseria gonorrhoeae, Haemophilus influenzae, Streptococcus pneumoniae, Streptococcus mutans and Helicobacter pylori*) provides a substantial benefit by allowing repair of DNA damage.

As discussed above in section 3, certain archaebacteria, namely *Halobacterium volcanii* and *Sulfolobus solfataricus,* appear to have distinctive mating systems involving DNA transfer through direct contacts between cells. We suggested that such mating systems may represent an intermediate stage in the transition from prokaryotic transformation to eukaryotic sex. In agreement with this view, Gross and Bhattacharya (2010) proposed that eukaryotic meiosis arose from archael conjugation and that both processes serve the same purpose, repair of damage, particularly double-strand breaks. These authors also suggested a model for restructuring of the archael cell during premeiotic evolution.

http://dx.doi.org/10.5772/56557

9. The adaptive function of transformation is likely repair of stress-induced DNA damage

Competence for transformation is induced specifically by DNA damaging conditions. For instance, the DNA damaging agents mitomycin C (a DNA interstrand cross-linking agent) and the fluoroquinolones norfloxacin, levofloxacin and moxifloxacin (topoisomerase inhibitors that causes double-strand breaks) induce transformation in *Streptococcus pneumoniae* (Claverys et al., 2006). Engelmoer and Rozen (2011) also showed, in *Streptococcus pneumoniae*, that transformation protects against the bactericidal effect of mitomycin C. In addition, induction of competence protects against the antibiotics streptomycin and kanamycin (Claverys et al., 2006; Engelmoer and Rozen, 2011). Although these aminoglycosides were, until recently, regarded as non-DNA damaging, work by Foti et al. (2012) in *Escherichia coli* suggests that a substantial portion of aminoglycoside bactericidal activity results from release of the hydroxyl radical (OH•) and induction of DNA damages including double-strand breaks.

DNA damaging UV irradiation increases transformation in *Bacillus subtilis* (Michod et al., 1988). Ciprofloxacin, which interacts with DNA gyrase and introduces double-strand breaks, induces expression of competence genes in *Helicobacter pylori*, thus enhancing the frequency of transformation (Dorer et al., 2010). Charpentier et al. (2011) tested 64 toxic molecules to determine which of these induce competence in *Legionella pneumophila*. Only six of these, all DNA damaging agents, caused strong induction. These agents were mitomycin C (which causes DNA inter-strand crosslinks), norfloxacin, ofloxacin and nalidixic acid [inhibitors of DNA gyrase that cause double-strand breaks (Albertini et al., 1995)], bicyclomycin [causes double-strand breaks (Washburn and Gottesman, 2011)], and hydroxyurea [causes oxidation of DNA bases (Sakano et al., 2001)]. UV irradiation also induced competence for transformation in *Legionella pneumophila*. Charpentier et al. (2011) suggested that competence for transformation probably evolved as a response to DNA damage.

The number of genome copies in logarithmically growing bacteria typically differ from the number of genomes in stationary phase bacteria, and this has implications for the capability of bacteria to carry out homologous recombinational repair (HRR). During logarithmic growth, two or more copies of any particular region of the chromosome are ordinarily present in a bacterial cell, as cell division is not precisely matched with chromosome replication. HRR is effective at repairing double-strand damages, such as double-strand breaks. This repair process depends on interaction of the damaged chromosome with a second homologous chromosome. During logarithmic growth, a DNA damage in one chromosome may be repaired by HRR using sequence information from the other homologous daughter chromosome. As bacterial cells approach stationary phase they typically have just one copy of the chromosome, and HRR requires input of an homologous template from another cell by transformation (Bernstein et al., 2012).

A series of experiments were carried out using *Bacillus subtilis* irradiated by UV light as the damaging agent to test whether the adaptive function of transformation is repair of DNA damages (for review, see Michod et al., 2008). The results of these experiments indicated that transforming DNA acts to repair potentially lethal DNA damages introduced by UV in the recipient DNA. The particular process responsible for repair was likely HRR.

In *Nisseria gonorrhoeae,* uptake of DNA during transformation depends on the presence of specific short nucleotide sequences (9-10mers residing in coding regions) in the donor DNA. These nucleotide sequences are called DNA uptake sequences (DUSs). DUSs occur at a particularly high density within genes involved in DNA repair, including HRR (Davidsen et al., 2004). Stohl and Seifert (2006) presented evidence that HRR mediated by the RecA protein plays an important role in protecting *Neisseria gonorrhoeae* against oxidative damage. Davidsen et al. (2004) suggested that the over-representation of DUSs in DNA repair genes may reveal the benefits of maintaining or restoring the integrity of the repair machinery through preferential uptake of genome maintenance genes that are especially important, and must be replaced by new copies if irreparably damaged or lost.

10. The sexual cycle is induced by stress in single-celled and simple multicellular eukaryotes

In eukaryotic microorganisms, sex occurs under stressful conditions as it does in bacteria. Among currently existing unicellular and simple multicellular eukaryotes, sexual reproduction is ordinarily facultative. These organisms usually reproduce asexually in a favorable environment, but reproduce sexually when under stress. Sex is induced in these organisms by starvation, mechanical damage, desiccation and heat shock. One example is the paramecium tetrahymena that can be induced to undergo conjugation (sexual mating) by starvation (Elliott and Hayes, 1953). Another example is the unicellular green alga *Chlamydomonas reinhardi*. When this organism is grown in a medium depleted of a source of nitrogen, vegetative cells differentiate into gametes (Sager & Granik, 1954). These gametes are then able to fuse, form zygotes and undergo meiosis. A further example is the haploid fission yeast *Schizosaccharomyces pombe*. This yeast is a facultative sexual microorganism that can undergo mating when nutrients become limiting (Davey, 1998). The budding yeast *Saccharomyces cerevisiae* reproduces by mitosis as diploid cells when nutrients are abundant. However, when starved, this yeast undergoes meiosis to form haploid spores (Herskowitz, 1988). The oomycete *Phytophthora cinnamomi* is induced to undergo sexual reproduction by hydrogen peroxide or mechanical damage to hyphae (Reeves and Jackson, 1974). Sex, in the multicellular green algae *Volvox carteri*, is induced by heat shock (Kirk and Kirk, 1986).

11. Meiosis is induced by DNA damaging conditions in microbial eukaryotes

In sections 2 and 5, above, we reviewed evidence that sex was present early in the evolution of eukaryotes, raising the likelihood that eukaryotic sex arose from ancestral prokaryotic sex. We also reviewed evidence in section 9 that bacterial sex (transformation) is an adaptation for

http://dx.doi.org/10.5772/56557

repair of DNA damages. In this section we present evidence that sex in eukaryotes, particularly the meiotic stage of the sexual cycle, is also an adaptation for response to DNA damage.

Hydrogen peroxide produces oxidative stress that causes a variety of DNA damages including modified bases and single- and double-strand breaks (Slupphang et al., 2003). When the yeast *Schizosaccharomyces pombe* was exposed to the oxidizing agent hydrogen peroxide, sex was induced (Bernstein and Johns, 1989). Mating and formation of sexual spores was increased by 4- to 18-fold upon exposure to hydrogen peroxide.

As mentioned in the preceding section, sex in the green algae *Volvox carterei* is induced by heat shock (Kirk and Kirk, 1986). This induction of sex is inhibited by anti-oxidants, indicating that heat shock induction of sex is mediated by oxidative stress (Nedelcu and Michod, 2003). Furthermore, Nedelcu et al. (2004) showed that an inhibitor of the mitochondrial electron transport chain, that induces oxidative stress, also induced sex in *Volvox carteri*. On the basis of this evidence Nedelcu and Michod (2003; 2004) suggested that reactive oxygen species produced by oxidative stress cause DNA damage leading to the induction of sex in *Volvox carteri*. Thus sex in *Volvox carterei*, as in *Schizosaccharomyces pombe*, appears to be an adaptation for coping with DNA damage induced by oxidative stress.

12. Recombinational repair of DNA damages in the germ line

Studies from a wide range of eukaryotes indicate that meiotic recombinational repair is an adaptation for repairing germ-line DNA damages. For example, exposure of eukaryotes to a DNA damaging agent causes increased meiotic recombination (expected as a result of HRR) as measured by exchange of allelic markers. Thus X-irradiation increases meiotic allelic recombination in *Saccharomyces cerevisiae* (Kelly et al., 1983) and in the nematode *Caenorhabditis elegans* (Kim and Rose, 1987). In the fruit fly *Drosophila melanogaster*, meiotic recombination is increased by UV light (Prudhommeau and Proust, 1973), gamma-rays (Suzuki and Parry, 1964) and mitomycin C (Schewe et al., 1971). These observations indicate that DNA damage increases homologous recombinational repair of the damage and this can be detected as increased allelic recombination.

In another type of experiment, Preston et al. (2006) studied the repair of double-strand breaks in the male germ line of *Drosophila* by the three repair processes of NHEJ (non-homologous end joining), SSA (single-strand annealing) and HR-h (homologous recombinational repair between non-sister homologs). They found that HR-h increased linearly in the germ line from 14% in young individuals to 60% in old ones, whereas the other pathways showed a corresponding decrease. The following explanation was offered for these findings. NHEJ and SSA are considered to be faster than HR-h and require no homologous template, but they are much more error-prone. Therefore NHEJ and SSA repair would be favored under conditions where the benefit of rapid gamete production outweighs the longer-term costs of inaccurate repair of DNA damage. The few individuals who survive to old age may occupy a less crowded environment where competition is decreased and opportunities to mate are rare. Under these conditions, the advantages of speed are negated and accurate HR-h repair becomes the favored strategy.

In some protozoans, vitality declines over the course of successive asexual cell divisions by binary fission. However, if sexual interaction (conjugation) occurs, vitality is restored. Evidence indicates that meiosis leads to rejuvination, and that this rejuvenation is associated with removal of DNA damages. The ciliate protozoan *Paramecium tetraurelia* has a polyploid macronucleus that contains about 800 to 1500 copies of the genome, and a diploid micronucleus. The macronuclear DNA expresses cellular functions, and the micronucleus contains the germline DNA. *Paramecium tetraurelia* is a facultative sexual microorganism that can reproduce asexually by binary fission or by a sexual process involving meiosis. There are two kinds of meiotic process; the first is a kind of outcrossing sex called conjugation, and the second is a kind of self-fertilization called automixis. In the asexual growth phase, during which cell divisions are by mitosis rather than meiosis, a gradual loss of vitality occurs that is referred to as clonal aging. If an asexual line of clonally aging paramecia fails to undergo conjugation or automixis it will die out after about 200 fissions.

Auferheide (1987) clarified the cause of clonal aging in *Paramecium tetraurelia* by the use of transplantation experiments. When macronuclei of clonally young paramecia were injected into clonally older paramecia, the lifespan of the older recipients was prolonged. In contrast, when cytoplasm, rather than macronuclei, was transplanted from young to older paramecia the lifespan of the recipients was not prolonged. These experiments suggested that clonal lifespan is determined by the macronucleus rather than the cytoplasm. Subsequent experiments by Smith-Sonneborn (1979), Holmes and Holmes (1986) and Gilley and Blackburn (1994) demonstrated that clonal aging is associated with a dramatic increase in DNA damage. When clonally aged paramecia undergo meiosis, either in association with conjugation or automixis, the old macronucleus disintegrates and a new macronucleus is formed by replication of the micronuclear DNA that had just experienced meiosis followed by fertilization. These paramecia were rejuvenated in the sense of having a restored clonal lifespan. It thus appears that clonal aging is caused, in large part, by a progressive increase in DNA damage; and that rejuvination is due to repair of these damages in the micronucleus during meiosis and the reestablishment of the macronucleus by replication of the newly repaired micronuclear DNA.

A similar phenomenon to clonal aging in paramecium is also found in yeast. In the budding yeast *Saccharomyes cerevisiae*, mother cells give rise to progeny buds by mitotic division. Mother cells undergo replicative aging over successive generations and, ultimately, death. However when a mother cell undergoes meiosis and gametogenesis, lifespan is reset (Unal et al., 2011). The replicative potential of gametes (spores) formed by aged cells is the same as gametes formed by young cells, indicating that age-associated damage is removed from the aged mother cells. This observation suggests that during meiosis removal of age-associated damages leads to rejuvination, but it is not yet clear if these damages are actually in the DNA.

In the nematode *Caenorhabditis elegans*, oocyte nuclei in the pachytene stage of meiosis (the stage in which recombination occurs between non-sister homologs) are hyper-resistant to X-irradiation compared to oocytes in diakinesis (a later stage of meiosis) or early embryonic cells after fertilization (Takanami et al., 2000). Pachytene hyper-resistance depends on expression of gene *ce-rdh-51*, a homolog of yeast gene *rad51* (*recA*-like) that catalyzes key steps in homologous recombinational repair. Furthermore, nuclei in the pachytene stage have greater resistance to heavy ion particle irradiation than nuclei in the later diplotene and diakinesis stages of meiosis, as well as nuclei in early embryonic cells (Takanami et al., 2003). Resistance during pachytene to heavy ion particle irradiation in *Caenorhabditis elegans* also depends on expression of gene *ce-rdh-51*, a *rad51/recA* homolog. In addition, this resistance also depends on gene *ce-atl-1*, a gene related to *atm* that is necessary for repair of double-strand breaks by homologous recombinational repair in mammals, and for fertility in mice and humans (Table 1). These observations indicate that *Caenorhabditis elegans* meiotic pachytene nuclei efficiently repair X-ray and heavy ion-induced DNA damage by homologous recombinational repair.

Coogan and Rosenblum (1988) measured the repair of double-strand damages after γ-irradiation of rat spermatogenic cells in sequential stages of germ cell formation (i.e. spermatagonia, preleptotene spermatocytes, pachytene spermatocytes and spermatid spermatocytes). The greatest repair capability occurred in pachytene spermatocytes, the meiotic stage in which recombinational repair occurs. These findings suggest that a function of meiosis, expressed during the pachytene stage, is the repair of double-strand damages. The most likely natural sources of the double-strand damages normally repaired at pachytene are reactive oxygen species generated by active metabolism.

Recombinational repair of DNA damages during meiosis also likely occurs in plants and depends on *rad51*, a *recA* ortholog. In *Arabidopsis thaliana*, mutants defective in a *rad51* paralog, *xrcc3*, are deficient in meiotic recombination and are sterile; they are also hypersensitive to mitomycin C, a DNA cross-linking agent (Bleuyard and White, 2004; Bleuyard et al., 2005). In rice (Oryza sativa), the *rad51C* gene is required for meiosis of both female and male gametocytes, and mutants deficient in this gene have increased sensitivity in somatic cells to the DNA alkylating agent methyl methanesulfonate and the cross-linking agent mitomycin C (Kou et al., 2012). In maize, mutants defective in homologs of *rad51* are deficient in meiosis and are sterile; they also produce embryos that are highly susceptible to induction of double-strand breaks by radiation (Li et al., 2007).

The observations summarized in this section imply that meiosis is an adaptation for recombinational repair of DNA damages in the germ line.

13. Unrepaired DNA damage during mammalian gametogenesis causes infertility

In mammals, germ cells are exposed to natural causes of DNA damage. For instance, several germ cell stages, including pachytene spermatocytes, have the potential to produce levels of reactive oxygen species sufficient to cause oxidative stress (Fisher and Atkin, 1997). Reactive oxygen species can produce double-strand damages in DNA. Also, heat can cause DNA damage. Paul et al. (2008) showed that mild heat stress (40 or 42ºC for 30 minutes) applied to the mouse scrotum causes DNA strand breaks in germ cells leading to infertility and abnormalities in embryonic development of progeny.

In the US, about 15% of all couples are infertile. A major cause of male infertility is oxidative stress during gametogenesis (Makker et al., 2009). Oxidative stress causes a variety of DNA damages including oxidized and ring fragmented bases and single- and double-strand breaks (Slupphang et al., 2003). Nili et al. (2011) showed that subfertile men have an increased frequency of sperm chromosomal aneuploidy as well as increased DNA damage (i.e. DNA strand breaks and alkali labile sites). Lewis and Aitken (2005) reviewed evidence that an increased level of DNA damage in the germ line of men is associated with poor semen quality, low rate of fertilization, impaired pre-implantation development, increased abortion, and a higher incidence of disease in progeny including childhood cancer. These authors also noted that the natural causes of this elevated DNA damage are unclear, but that the principal candidate is oxidative stress.

Genes whose products are employed in recombinational repair (e.g. *atm, brca1, dmc1, mlh1, pms2, mlh5 and ercc1*) are expressed at a substantially higher level in testes than in somatic cells of males, and inherited mutations in these genes cause infertility (Table 1).

Genetic defect	Mutant female and/or male infertility	Expression in testes of the wild-type gene	References
atm$^{(+/-)}$	Females and males in both mice and humans are infertile	4-fold increased mRNA expression in human testes vs. somatic cells	Barlow et al., 1998; Galetzka et al., 2007
brca1$^{(-/-)}$	The few surviving male mice are infertile	3-fold increased mRNA expression in human testes vs. somatic cells	Cressman et al., 1999; Galetzka et al., 2007
dmc1$^{(-/-)}$	Female and male mice are infertile; *dmc*$^{(+/-)}$ women undergo premature ovarian failure	Expression specific for meiotic cells	Pittman et al., 1998; Mandon-Pepin et al., 2008
mlh1$^{(-/-)}$	Female and male mice are infertile	1.7-fold increased mRNA expression in human testes vs. somatic cells	Wei et al., 2002; Galetzka et al., 2007
pms2$^{(+/-)}$ or *pms2*$^{(-/-)}$	Male infertility and sperm DNA damage	2 to 4-fold increased mRNA expression in human testes vs. somatic cells	Galetzka et al., 2007; Ji et al., 2012
msh5$^{(-/-)}$	Female and male *msh5*$^{(-/-)}$ mice are infertile; women who are *msh5*$^{(+/-)}$ or *msh5*$^{(-/-)}$ undergo premature ovarian failure	Expression specific for meiotic cells	Edelmann et al., 1999; Mandon-Pepin et al., 2008
ercc1$^{(-/-)}$	Female and male mice are infertile	Expressed at a high level in mouse testes	Hsia et al. (2003)

Table 1. The effect on fertility of mutations in genes employed in meiotic recombinational repair and the increased expression of these genes in testes

In humans, the mismatch repair genes *mlh1*, *pms2* and *msh5* participate in meiotic recombination. Variants of these genes that are common in human populations cause increased risk of male infertility (Ji et al., 2012). Also variants of *mlh1* and *pms2* cause increased sperm DNA damage.

In women, about half of fertilized eggs fail to produce embryos that survive, as is typical of mammals generally (Austin, 1972). Roberts and Lowe (1975) estimated that about half of all post-implantation embryos are lost, often before the first missed period. Also, Wilcox et al. (1988) noted that, after implantation, about 31% of embryos miscarry, often before the woman is aware that she is pregnant. Although the basis for these malfunctions is not yet established, it is likely that unrepaired DNA damage is an important contributing factor. Adriaens et al. (2009) reviewed several studies showing that the mammalian oocyte can repair various kinds of DNA damage occurring either spontaneously or as a consequence of exposure to external agents. However these repair processes are not 100% efficient.

Chemotherapy used in cancer treatment can result in infertility in young female cancer survivors. Soleimani et al. (2011) showed that exposure to the chemotherapeutic agent doxorubicin causes massive double-strand breaks in human and rodent oocytes leading to apoptotic cell death. Activation of the recombinational repair pathway appeared to allow only a minority of oocytes to survive.

The inheritance of a mutant *brca1* allele leading to heterozygosity [$brca1^{(+/-)}$] can dramatically increase a woman's life-time risk for developing breast cancer. The Brca1 protein has a key role in recombinational repair of DNA damages in somatic cells and in meiosis during oogenesis. Oktay et al. (2010) found that infertile women who are heterozygous for a *brca1* mutation do not respond well to clinical treatments for enhancing fertility. This finding suggested that deficiency of Brca1 mediated recombinational repair during oogenesis reduces fertility.

Reproductive capacity of women begins to diminish after young adulthood (i.e. about age 37 years). Recently, Titus et al. (2013) showed that DNA double-strand breaks – a measure of DNA damage – accumulate with age in primordial follicles (immature primary oocytes) of mice and humans. Paralleling this increase in breaks, expression of key recombinational repair genes *brca1*, *mre11*, *rad51* and *atm* declined in oocytes of mice and humans. In *brca1*-deficient mice [$brca1^{(+/-)}$], double-strand breaks increased, numbers of primordial follicles decreased and reproductive capacity declined relative to wild-type mice. Women with a *brca1* mutation were also found to have a lower ovarian reserve. Using RNA interference in mouse oocytes, it was found that inhibition of expression of *brca1*, *mre11*, *rad51* or *atm* increased double-strand breaks and decreased oocyte survival (Titus et al., 2013). These findings implicate deficient recombinational repair and consequent accumulation of DNA damages as important determinants of oocyte aging. Furthermore, Mandon-Pepin et al. (2008) showed that mutations in either of two genes that are active in meiotic recombinational repair (*dmc1* and *msh5*) are associated with loss of normal ovarian function in women younger than 40 years of age (Table 1).

The findings described in this section indicate that DNA damage during spermatogenesis and oogenesis can lead to infertility, a significant clinical problem for humans. Furthermore, meiotic recombinational repair likely plays an important role in repairing such DNA damages and avoiding infertility.

14. Homologous recombinational repair functions similarly during meiosis and mitosis, but has greater scope for repairing double-strand damages during meiosis

Homologous recombinational repair occurs during mitosis, but is largely limited to interaction between nearby sister-chromosomes subsequent to replication (but prior to cell division). During mitosis, the frequency of recombination between non-sister homologous chromosomes is only about 1% of that between sister-chromosomes (Moynahan and Jasin, 2010). In contrast, during meiosis, recombination between non-sister homologous chromosomes is frequent and is indeed a key characteristic of meiosis. Despite these differences concerning which homologous chromosomes are involved, the machinery of recombinational repair appears to be closely similar during mitosis and meiosis. Numerous common gene products are essential to both processes. The parallels in the machinery of recombinational repair across meiosis and mitosis in eukaryotes, and even extending to the mechanism of recombination during transformation in bacteria, suggests similarity of function.

In the budding yeast *Saccharomyces cerevisiae*, mutations in several genes needed for meiotic and mitotic recombination cause increased sensitivity to radiation and/or genotoxic chemicals (Haynes and Kunz, 1981). For instance, gene *rad52* is required for both meiotic recombination (Game et al., 1980) and mitotic recombination (Malone and Esposito, 1980). *Rad52* mutants have increased sensitivity to killing by X-rays, methylmethane sulfonate and the DNA cross-linking agent 8-methoxypsoralen-plus-UV light, and show reduced meiotic recombination (Haynes and Kunz, 1981; Henriques and Moustacchi, 1980; Game et al., 1980), suggesting that recombinational repair is needed for the repair of the different DNA damages caused by these agents.

Mutants of the fruit fly *Drosophila melanogaster* that are defective in the "meiotic genes" *mei-41* and *mei-9* have increased sensitivity to X-rays, UV, methylmethane sulfonate, nitrogen mustard, benzo(s)pyrene and 2-acetylaminofluorene, and are also defective in meiotic recombination (Baker et al., 1976; Boyd, 1978; Rasmusen, 1984). In addition, mutants defective in genes *hdm* and *DmRad51/spnA* are deficient in meiotic recombination and also have increased sensitivity to X-rays or methylmethane sulfonate, (Joyce et al., 2009; Staeva-Viera et al., 2003) suggesting a deficiency in recombinational repair in somatic cells. *Drosophila* mutants defective in *brca2* are also deficient in both meiotic and mitotic recombinational repair (Klovstad et al., 2008). Overall, mutants of *Drosophila* that are defective in genes essential for carrying out recombination (i.e. genes *mei-41*, *mei-9*, *hdm*, *spnA* and *brca2*) are more sensitive to killing by a variety of DNA damaging agents than are wild-type flies. This increased sensitivity is likely caused by a reduced capability of the somatic cells of the flies to perform recombinational repair of the DNA damages caused by these agents. These same mutants also

http://dx.doi.org/10.5772/56557

have reduced meiotic recombination, indicating that they are likely deficient in homologous recombinational repair of DNA damages during meiosis.

Homologous recombinational repair during meiosis provides a unique advantage compared to mitosis. During meiosis, systematic pairing and recombination between non-sister homologous chromosomes is promoted compared to mitosis, where recombination between non-sisters chromosomes is infrequent (Moynahan and Jasin, 2010). Consequently, during mitosis, homologous recombinational repair is largely restricted to the portion of the cell cycle in which DNA replication is occurring (S phase) and after DNA replication is complete (G2 phase) so that a closely adjacent homologous chromosome is available. During this restricted period of the mitotic cell cycle, double-strand damages may be accurately removed by homologous recombinational repair between sister homologs (Tichy et al., 2010). However, during the portion of the mitotic cell cycle after cell division but prior to DNA replication (G1 phase), double-strand damages, such as double-strand breaks and interstrand crosslinks, are not ordinarily repaired by accurate homologous recombinational repair. Rather, they are either repaired by the inaccurate process of non-homologous end-joining that generates mutation, or else the double-strand damages cause cell death.

In contrast to the constraint on DNA repair during mitosis, during meiosis, homologous recombinational repair can accurately remove double-strand damages that arise at any stage of the cell cycle because of systematic pairing of non-sister homologous chromosomes. Cells in the G1 phase of meiosis are more resistant to the lethal effects of X-rays than cells in the G1 phase of mitosis (Kelley et al., 1983). This finding suggests that types of damages caused by X-rays, which include double-strand damages, are more readily repaired during meiotic G1 than mitotic G1. Repair capability during meiosis is likely more effective than during mitosis, because there is greater access to a homolog for the source of needed redundant information and also because the proteins that catalyze homologous recombinational repair are present at an increased level (Table 1).

In this section we reviewed evidence that DNA damages caused by a variety of exogenous agents are repaired by homologous recombinational repair during mitosis. Since this repair process is closely similar to the analogous process during meiosis, we infer that homologous recombination during meiosis also functions to repair a variety of DNA damages.

During each cell cycle in humans, 30,000 to 50,000 DNA replication origins are activated (Mechali, 2010). Thus chromosomes are replicated in segments. During pre-meiotic replication, a double-strand damage in any segment may block completion of replication of the segment until the damage is repaired. During the subsequent prophase I stage of meiosis when the blocked segment becomes paired with a non-sister homolog, the damage may be accurately repaired by recombinational repair using the intact information from the non-sister homolog. After the damage is removed, replication of the segment can be completed. Hence meiosis can provide a means for accurately repairing double-strand damages present in all stages of the preceding cell cycle.

15. The key role of RecA repair protein in bacterial transformation

In this section we focus on the role of the RecA protein and its orthologs in catalyzing key steps of recombination during transformation. First, RecA interacts with ATP and single-stranded DNA to form a helical filament. This filament then binds to double-stranded DNA, searches for homology and next catalyses exchange with the complementary strand of the duplex DNA producing a new heteroduplex (Chen et al., 2008). Pairing of homologous regions of the two parental genomes leads to exchange of information between the genomes (recombination).

The RecA protein is essential for transformation in the bacteria *Bacillus subtilis, Streptococcus pneumoniae* and *Neisseria gonorrhoeae* (Dubnau et al., 1973; Martin et al., 1992; Claverys et al., 2009; Stohl et al., 2011). In *Streptococcus pneumoniae* expression of the *recA* gene is induced during development of competence (Mortier-Barriere et al., 1998). In *Bacillus subtilis*, expression of the *recA* gene is induced following DNA damage, as well as during development of the competent state (Cheo et al., 1992).

In *Bacillus subtilis* transformation, the RecA protein first interacts with several other competence proteins to form a multiprotein complex. This complex next interacts with incoming single-stranded DNA at a cell pole to prepare the entering DNA for recombination with the resident chromosome (Kidane and Graumann, 2005). The interaction of the single-stranded DNA with RecA protein leads to formation of striking filamentous structures that emanate from the cell pole harboring the competence machinery, and then extend further into the cytosol. Kidane and Graumann (2005) considered that these RecA/single-stranded DNA filamentous threads represent dynamic nucleofilaments that scan the chromosome for regions of homology. By this process, incoming DNA is brought to the homologous site in the bacterial chromosome where informational exchange occurs.

The molecular interactions of bacterial RecA protein with DNA were analyzed by Cox (1991; 1993) who concluded the RecA protein evolved as the central component of an homologous recombinational repair system for dealing with DNA damage. Cox concluded that DNA repair is the most important function of homologous genetic recombination. This conclusion is in accord with the idea that, in bacterial transformation, RecA protein functions to remove DNA damages in the resident chromosome by homologous recombinational repair using intact (undamaged) information from the donor chromosome. As noted above, bacteria typically become competent for transformation in late log phase, when most cells are haploid and the only available source of intact homologous DNA is another bacterium.

16. The key role of RecA orthologs in eukaryotic meiosis

In this section we present evidence that orthologs of the RecA protein have a similar role in eukaryotic meiosis to that in bacterial transformation, the facilitation of recombinational repair between two homologous DNA molecules of different parental origin.

Protein components of the homologous recombination machinery appear to be highly conserved from bacteria to eukaryotes. We first consider unicellular, and then multicellular eukaryotes. Genes *rad51* and *dmc1* of the yeasts *Saccharomyces cerevisiae* and *Schizosaccharomyces pombe* are orthologs of the bacterial *recA* gene. The tertiary structure of the yeast Dmc1 recombinase is similar to the overall structure of the bacterial RecA recombinase (Story et al., 1993). In addition to yeast, the *dmc1* gene has also been identified in other unicellular eukaryotes, i.e. *Giardia, Trypanosoma, Leishmania, Entamoeba* and *Plasmodium* (Ramesh et al., 2005). The yeast Rad51 and Dmc1 proteins interact with single-stranded DNA to form a presynaptic filament that initiates recombinational repair (Sauvageau et al., 2005; San Filippo et al., 2008). This filament is similar to the RecA/single-stranded DNA nucleofilament, described above, that is formed during bacterial transformation. Whereas the Dmc1 recombinase only acts during meiosis, Rad51 acts both during meiosis and mitosis (Bugreev et al., 2011). Thus the Rad51 and Dmc1 recombinases that perform key steps in meiosis of unicellular eukaryotes appear to be structurally and functionally similar to the bacterial RecA recombinase that performs key steps of transformation in bacteria. This similarity suggests evolution of the sexual process of meiosis from the sexual process of transformation.

We next review evidence that orthologs of bacterial RecA play a key role in meiotic recombination in multicellular animals and plants, suggesting evolutionary continuity of the central role of recA orthologs in sexual processes from microorganisms to multicellular life forms.

Orthologs of the RecA protein play a key role in meiosis of animals (e.g. nematodes, mice and humans) and of plants (e.g. *Arabidopsis*, rice and lilies). In the nematode *Caenorhabditis elegans,* resistance to X-ray induced DNA damage in meiotic pachytene nuclei depends on the strongly expressed *recA*-like gene (*ce-rdh-1*) (Takenami et al., 2000), implying a key role of this gene in meiotic recombinational repair.

In the testis and ovary of the mouse, a homolog of the *recA* and *rad51* genes is expressed at a high level, suggesting that a RecA-like protein is employed in meiotic recombination in the mouse (Shinohara et al., 1993). In the mouse, mutations in the *dmc1* gene, which encodes the meiosis specific recombinase, cause an inability to complete meiosis, failure to undergo intimate pairing of homologous chromosomes, and sterility (Pittman et al., 1998; Yoshida et al., 1998; see Table 1). In humans, Dmc1 recombinase forms nucleoprotein complexes with single-stranded DNA that promote the search for homology and informational exchange reactions that are crucial steps of recombinational repair (Sehorn et al., 2004; Bugreev et al., 2005).

Rad51 and Dmc1, RecA-like recombinases, are required for meiosis in the plant *Arabidopsis thaliana* (Li et al., 2004; Couteau et al., 1999). In the lily, Rad51 and Lim15 (an ortholog of Dmc1) co-localize on meiotic prophase I chromosomes where they form discrete foci (Terasawa et al., 1995). The proteins of these foci are though to cooperate in the search for homology and the pairing of homologous sequences. Similarly, in rice an ortholog of Dmc1 promotes the pairing of homologous chromosomes and is required for meiosis (Deng and Wang, 2007).

17. Another key repair protein employed in both transformation and meiosis

Prior to the assembly of the RecA recombinase or an equivalent ortholog recombinase on single-stranded DNA to form a presynaptic filament, a single-strand-binding protein [termed SSB in bacteria and RPA (replication protein A) in eukaryotes], processes the single-stranded DNA. *Bacillus subtilis* and *Streptococcus pneumoniae* encode a single-stranded DNA binding protein (SsbB) that is expressed uniquely during competence for genetic transformation, and directly protects internalized donor single-stranded DNA (Attaiech et al., 2011). In *Streptococcus pneumoniae,* SsbB is highly abundant, and potentially could allow the binding of half a genome equivalent of DNA (Attaiech et al., 2011). SsbB participates in the processing of ssDNA into recombinants, and is of crucial importance for chromosomal transformation. Thus, in both transformation and meiosis, recombination depends on an analogous accessory protein, in addition to the RecA and RecA-like recombinases.

18. Meiosis, sex and outcrossing

The essential feature of meiosis is information exchange between two genomic DNA molecules derived from different individuals (parents). This feature is shared with bacterial transformation, which we have proposed here to be the ancestral precursor to meiosis. The two different individuals that participate in mating events leading to meiosis may be closely or distantly related to each other. When the two individuals are distantly related to each other they are likely to differ more genetically than if closely related. Thus in matings of distantly related individuals there is a greater potential for generating genetically varied progeny than in matings of closely related individuals.

Evolutionary biologists have often assumed that the potential benefit of producing genetically varied progeny is of substantially greater consequence than the advantage of DNA repair and is, by itself, sufficient to explain the adaptive advantage of meiosis specifically, and the adaptive benefit of sex generally. Critical evaluations of this view have been presented elsewhere (e.g. Bernstein et al., 1987; Birdsell & Wills, 2003; Michod et al., 2008; Gorelick & Heng, 2011; Horandl, 2009; Horandl, this volume). However, our view, in brief, is that genetic variation is a byproduct of homologous recombinational repair during meiosis, and that any benefit of producing varied progeny is a long-term population level effect that would supplement the advantage of DNA repair. DNA repair is an immediate benefit that occurs at each sexual generation. In the short term, the benefit of variation, we think, is unlikely to be adequate, by itself, to maintain sex, especially in those organisms where the costs of sex are high (see Michod et al., 2008; Horandl, this volume).

In many microbial eukaryotes, it is likely that, in nature, mating occurs most often between members of the same clonal population and that outcrossing is uncommon. For instance, Ruderfer et al. (2006) analyzed the ancestry of natural yeast *Saccharomyces cereviae* strains and concluded that outcrossing occurs only about once every 50,000 cell divisions. Mating is almost always between closely related yeast cells in nature. Mating occurs when haploid yeast cells of opposite mating type MATa and MATα come into contact. Zeyl and Otto (2007) and Ruderfer et al. (2006) pointed out that such contacts are frequent between closely related yeast cells for two reasons. The first reason is that cells of opposite mating type are present together in close proximity in the same ascus (an ascus is the sac that contains the cells directly produced by a single meiosis). The second reason for frequent contact between closely related cells is that haploid *Saccharomyces cerevisiae* cells of one mating type, upon cell division, often produce daughter cells of the opposite mating type. Thus, in this yeast, it appears that under natural conditions meiotic events that produce negligible recombinational variation are vastly more common than meiotic events that do produce variation. The relative rarity of meiotic events that result from outcrossing and produce recombinational variation is consistent with the idea that the main adaptive function of meiosis is recombinational repair of DNA damage, since this benefit is realized at each meiosis whether or not outcrossing occurs. Furthermore it is difficult to comprehend how meiosis, a complex developmental process, could be maintained through natural selection during the 50,000 cell divisions between outcrossing events, if the primary benefit of meiosis were production of genetic variation.

Among early facultatively sexual eukaryotes, the requirement of sex that two different parental genomes come together in a common cytoplasm would have led to a brief diploid interval. However, these early facultatively sexual organisms were likely primarily haploid, reproducing asexually as haploid organisms and only experiencing diploidy transiently during sex. As eukaryotes evolved further, the diploid stage of the life cycle became more extended, and eventually became predominant as in present day mammals and higher plants. As the diploid stage increased in importance, outcrossing also became more important because genomes of distantly related individuals are less likely than genomes of related individuals to contain common mutations. Thus outcrossing allows the masking of expression of deleterious recessive mutations in the diploid stage (Bernstein et al., 1985; Bernstein et al., 1987; Birdsell and Wills, 2003). The mutual masking of deleterious recessive mutations is referred to as complementation, a phenomenon underlying such concepts as hybrid vigor, heterosis, avoidance of inbreeding depression, and the incest taboo. We consider that these advantages of outcrossing are secondary benefits of sexual reproduction that arose with the development of a significant diploid stage, and that the primary advantage has remained homologous recombinational repair of damages in the DNA to be passed on to progeny.

19. Summary and conclusions

In bacteria, transformation involves transfer of DNA from a donor bacterial cell to a recipient cell, and can be regarded as a primitive form of sex. Competence for transformation arises by a complex developmental process that requires expression of numerous bacterial genes. Therefore competence appears to be an evolved adaptation that is of substantial benefit to the bacterium. Competence ordinarily develops during exposure to stressful environmental conditions such as growth to high cell density and nutritional limitation. Such stress conditions tend to cause increased DNA damage. Studies of transformation in several different bacterial species indicate that transformation is an adaptive response to DNA damage, and that it functions to repair DNA through the process of homologous recombinational repair.

Eukaryotes emerged in evolution from prokaryotic ancestors over 1.5 billion years ago. Based on recent evidence, meiosis, and thus sexual reproduction, appears to have arisen very early in the evolution of eukaryotes. Transformation and meiotic sex both involve the coming together of DNA molecules from separate individuals, recombination between these molecules, and passage of the recombined DNA to progeny. Thus transformation and meiosis are similar at a fundamental level. This similarity suggests that meiotic sex evolved from ancestral prokaryotic sex, that is, from bacterial transformation. In extant eukaryotic microorganisms sex is generally facultative and tends to occur under stressful conditions that are similar to the conditions that induce competence for transformation in bacteria. Also in extant eukaryotic microorganisms, sex is induced by agents that cause DNA damage. Damage to the genome (DNA in most species) appears to be a fundamental problem for life. In multicellular eukaryotes, defective recombinational repair during meiosis causes infertility that is likely due to accumulation of excessive DNA damages.

The RecA protein catalyzes key steps in recombination during bacterial transformation. Orthologs of RecA (e.g. Rad51 and Dmc1 proteins) in eukaryotes catalyze similar steps in recombination during meiosis. The RecA protein and its orthologs interact with single-stranded DNA to form a presynaptic nucleofilament that initiates recombination. This nucleofilament is thought to scan the partner chromosome for regions of homology in preparation for the informational exchange reactions of homologous recombinational repair. Other proteins that interact with the RecA protein or its orthologs also seem to carry out similar functions in transformation and meiosis. These similarities in the machinery of recombinational repair during transformation and meiosis suggest continuity in the evolution of sexual processes through the prokaryote to eukaryote boundry.

As the early eukaryotes evolved from their prokaryote ancestors, the diploid phase of the sexual cycle became increasingly prominent compared to the haploid phase. With the increasing prominence of diploidy, avoidance of expression of deleterious recessive mutations in diploid cells became advantageous. The two individuals that participate in a mating may be either distantly or closely related. A consequence of outcrossing, the mating of distantly related individuals, is that deleterious recessive mutations occurring in one parent are not likely to occur in the other, and so the expression of deleterious mutations tend to be masked in the progeny's diploid cells. This mutual masking of deleterious recessive mutations is referred to as complementation, a phenomenon that underlies hybrid vigor. In contrast, closely related individual are likely to share the same deleterious recessive mutations, and matings between them are more likely to lead to expression of deleterious recessive mutations in progeny. Thus, adaptations have evolved to promote outcrossing. Outcrossing organisms are also more likely to produce genetically varied progeny than inbreeding individuals and this also may provide advantages over time at the population level.

http://dx.doi.org/10.5772/56557

Author details

Harris Bernstein and Carol Bernstein*

*Address all correspondence to: bernstein324@yahoo.com

Department of Cellular and Molecular Medicine, College of Medicine, University of Arizona, Tucson, Arizona, USA

References

[1] Adriaens, I., Smitz, J. & Jacquet, P. (2009). The current knowledge on radiosensitivity of ovarian follicle development stages. *Human Reproduction Update*, Vol. 15(3), pp. 359-377.

[2] Akamatsu, T. & Taguchi, H. (2001). Incorporation of the whole chromosomal DNA in protoplast lysates into competent cells of *Bacillus subtilis*. *Bioscience, Biotechnology, and Biochemistry*, Vol. 65(4), pp. 823-829.

[3] Akopyants, N.S., Kimblin, N., Secundino, N., Patrick, R., Peters, N., Lawyer, P., Dobson, D.E., Beverley, S.M. & Sacks, D.L. (2009). Demonstration of genetic exchange during cyclical development of *Leishmania* in the sand fly vector. *Science*, Vol. 324, pp. 265-268.

[4] Albertini, S., Chételat, A.A., Miller, B., Muster, W., Pujadas, E., Strobel, R. & Gocke, E. (1995). Genotoxicity of 17 gyrase- and four mammalian topoisomerase II-poisons in prokaryotic and eukaryotic test systems. *Mutagenesis*, Vol. 10(4), pp. 343-351.

[5] Ames, B.N., Shigenaga, M.K. & Hagen, T.M. (1993). Oxidants, antioxidants, and the degenerative diseases of aging. Proceedings of the National Academy of Sciences USA, Vol. 90(17), pp. 7915-7922.

[6] Anagnostopoulos, C. & Spizizen, J. (1961). Requirements for transformation in *Bacillus subtilis*. *Journal of Bacteriology*, Vol. 81, pp. 741-746.

[7] Aspiras, M.B., Ellen, R.P. & Cvitkovitch, D.G. (2004). ComX activity of *Streptococcus mutans* growing in biofilms. *FEMS Microbiology Letters*, Vol. 238(1), pp. 167-174.

[8] Attaiech, L., Olivier, A., Mortier-Barriere, I., Soulet, A.-L., Granadel, C., Martin, B., Polard, P. & Claverys, J.-P. (2011). Role of the single-stranded DNA-binding protein SsbB in *Pneumococcal* transformation: Maintenance of a reservoir for genetic plasticity. *PLoS Genetics*, Vol. 7(6), pp. 1-12.

[9] Aufderheide, K.J. (1987). Clonal aging in *Paramecium tetraurelia*. II. Evidence of functional changes in the macronucleus with age. *Mechanisms of Ageing and Development*, Vol. 37, pp. 265-279.

[10] Austin, C.R. (1972). Pregnancy losses and birth defects. In: Austin, C.R., Short, R.V. editors. Reproduction in Mammals. Book 2, Chapter 5, London: Cambridge University Press, p. 134.

[11] Baker, B.S., Boyd, J.B., Carpenter, A.T.C., Green, M.M., Nguyen, T.D., Ripoll, P. & Smith, P.D. (1976). Genetic controls of meiotic recombination and somatic DNA metabolism in Drosophila melanogaster. Proceedings of the National Academy of Sciences USA, Vol. 73(11), pp. 4140-4144.

[12] Barlow, C., Liyanage, M., Moens, P.B., Tarsounas, M., Nagashima, K., Brown, K., Rottinghaus, S., Jackson, S.P., Tagle, D., Ried, T. & Wynshaw-Boris, A. (1998). Atm deficiency results in severe meiotic disruption as early as leptonema of prophase I. Development, Vol. 125, pp. 4007-4017.

[13] Bell, J.C., Plank, J.L., Dombrowski, C.C. & Kowalczykowski, S.C. (2012). Direct imaging of RecA nucleation and growth on single molecules of SSB-coated ssDNA. Nature, Vol. 491(7423), pp. 274-278.

[14] Bernstein C., & Johns, V. (1989). Sexual reproduction as a response to H_2O_2 damage in *Schizosaccharomyces pombe. Journal of Bacteriology,* Vol. 171(4), pp. 1893-1897.

[15] Bernstein, C., Bernstein, H., Payne, C.M. & Garewal, H. (2002). DNA repair/pro-apoptotic dual-role proteins in five major DNA repair pathways: fail-safe protection against carcinogenesis. *Mutation Research,* Vol. 511, pp. 145-178.

[16] Bernstein, C & Bernstein, H. (2004). Aging and sex, DNA repair in. In: *Encyclopedia of Molecular Cell Biology and Molecular Medicine,* Vol. 1, R.A. Meyers, ed., pp. 53-98, Wiley-VCH, Weinheim.

[17] Bernstein H., Byerly, H.C., Hopf, F.A. & Michod, R.E. (1985). Genetic damage, mutation, and the evolution of sex. *Science,* Vol. 229, pp.1277-1281.

[18] Bernstein, H., Hopf, F.A. & Michod, R.E. (1987). The molecular basis of the evolution of sex. *Advances in Genetics,* Vol. 24, pp. 323-370.

[19] Bernstein, H. & Bernstein, C. (2010). Evolutionary origin of recombination during meiosis. *BioScience,* 60(7), 498-435.

[20] Bernstein, H., Bernstein, C. & Michod, R.E. (2011). Meiosis as an evolutionary adaptation for DNA repair. In: *DNA Repair,* Kruman, I., ed., InTech Publ. Rijeka, Croatia, Chapter 19, pp. 357-382.

[21] Bernstein, H., Bernstein C. & Michod, R.E. (2012). DNA repair as the primary adaptive function of sex in bacteria and eukaryotes. In: *DNA Repair: New Research.* Nova Science Publishers, New York, Chapter 1: pp. 1-49.

[22] Bertani, G. & Baresi, L. (1987). Genetic transformation in the methanogen *Methanococcus voltae* PS. *Journal of Bacteriology,* Vol. 169(6), pp. 2730-2738.

http://dx.doi.org/10.5772/56557

[23] Birdsell, J.A. & Wills, C. (2003). The evolutionary origin and maintenance of sexual recombination: A review of contemporary models. In: *Evolutionary Biology*. R.G. MacIntyre, M.T. Clegg, (Eds.), pp. 27-138. Kluwer Academic/Plenum Publishers.

[24] Bleuyard, J.Y. & White, C.I. (2004). The Arabidopsis homologue of Xrcc3 plays an essential role in meiosis. *The EMBO Journal*, Vol. 23, pp. 439-449.

[25] Bleuyard, J.Y., Gallego, M.E., Savigny, F. & White, C.I. (2005). Differing requirements for the Arabidopsis Rad51 paralogs in meiosis and DNA repair. *The Plant Journal*, Vol. 41, pp. 533-545.

[26] Boussau, B., Karlberg, E.O., Frank, A.C., Legault, B.A. & Andersson, S.G. (2004). Computational inference of scenarios for alpha-proteobacterial genome evolution. *Proceedings of the National Academy of Sciences USA*, Vol. 101(26), pp. 9722-9727.

[27] Boyd, J.B. (1978). DNA repair in *Drosophila*. In: Hanawalt, P.C., Friedberg, E.C., Fox, C.F., editors. *DNA Repair Mechanisms*. New York: Academic Press, pp. 449-452.

[28] Bray, C.M. & West, C.E. (2005). DNA repair mechanisms in plants: crucial sensors and effectors for the maintenance of genome integrity. *New Phytologist*, 168(3), pp. 511-528.

[29] Bugreev, D.V., Golub, E.I., Stasiak, A.Z., Stasiak, A. & Mazin, A.V. (2005). Activation of human meiosis-specific recombinase Dmc1 by Ca^{2+}. *Journal of Biological Chemistry*, Vol. 280(29), pp. 26886-26895.

[30] Bugreev, D.V., Pezza, R.J., Mazina, O.M., Voloshin, O.N., Camerini-Otero, R.D. & Mazin, A.V. (2011). The resistance of DMC1 D-loops to dissociation may account for the DMC1 requirement in meiosis. *Nature Structural and Molecular Biology*, Vol. 18(1), pp. 56-61.

[31] Butterfield, N.J. (2000). *Bangiomorpha pubescens* n. gen., n. sp.: implications for the evolution of sex, multicellularity, and the Mesoproterozoic/Neoproterozoic radiation of eukaryotes. *Paleobiology*, Vol. 26(3), pp. 386-404.

[32] Charpentier, X., Kay, E., Schneider, D., & Shuman, H.A. (2011). Antibiotics and UV radiation induce competence for natural transformation in *Legionella pneumophila*. *Journal of Bacteriology*, Vol. 193(5), pp. 1114-1121.

[33] Cheah, K.S.E. & Osborne, D.J. (1978). DNA lesions occur with loss of viability in embryos of ageing rye seed. *Nature*, Vol. 272, pp. 593-599.

[34] Chen, I. & Dubnau D. (2004). DNA uptake during bacterial transformation. *Nature Reviews/Microbiology*, Vol. 2(3), pp. 241-249.

[35] Chen, Z., Yang, H. & Pavletich, N.P. (2008). Mechanism of homologous recombination from RecA-ssDNA/dsDNA structures. *Nature*, Vol. 453, pp. 489-496.

[36] Cheo, D.L., Bayles, K.W. & Yasbin, R.E. (1992). Molecular characterization of regulatory elements controlling expression of the *Bacillus subtilis recA*$^+$ gene. *Biochimie*, Vol. 74, pp. 755-762.

[37] Claverys, J.P., Prudhomme, M. & Martin, B. (2006). Induction of competence regulons as a general response to stress in gram-positive bacteria. *Annual Review of Microbiology*, Vol. 60, pp. 451-475.

[38] Claverys, J.P., Martin, B., & Polard, P. (2009). The genetic transformation machinery: composition, localization and mechanism. *FEMS Microbiology Reviews*, Vol. 33, pp. 643-656.

[39] Cline, S.W., Schalkwyk, L.C. & Doolittle, W.F. (1989). Transformation of the archaebacterium *Halobacterium volcanii* with genomic DNA. *Journal of Bacteriology*, Vol. 171(9), pp. 4987-4991.

[40] Coogan, T.P. & Rosenblum, I.Y. (1988). DNA double-strand damage and repair following -irradiation in isolated spermatogenic cells. *Mutation Research*, Vol. 194, pp. 183-191.

[41] Cooper, M.A., Adam, R.D., Worobey, M. & Sterling, C.R. (2007). Population genetics provides evidence for recombination in *Giardia*. *Current Biology*, Vol. 17, pp. 1984-1988.

[42] Couteau, F., Belzile, F., Horlow, C., Grandjean, O., Vezon, D. & Doutriaux, M.P. (1999). Random chromosome segregation without meiotic arrest in both male and female meiocytes of a *dmc1* mutant of *Arabidopsis*. *The Plant Cell*, Vol. 11, pp. 1623-1634.

[43] Cox, C.J., Foster, P.G., Hirt, R.P., Harris, S.R. & Embley, T.M. (2008). The archaebacterial origin of eukaryotes. *Proceedings of the National Academy of Sciences USA*, Vol. 105(51), pp. 20356-20361.

[44] Cox, M.M. (1991). The RecA protein as a recombinational repair system. *Molecular Microbiology*, Vol. 5(6), pp. 1295-1299.

[45] Cox, M.M. (1993). Relating biochemistry to biology: How the recombinational repair function of RecA protein is manifested in its molecular properties. *BioEssays*, Vol. 15(9), 617-623.

[46] Cox, P.A. (1988). Hydrophilous pollination. *Annual Review of Ecology and Systematics*, Vol. 19, pp. 261-279.

[47] Cressman, V.L., Backlund, D.C., Avrutskaya, A.V., Leadon, S.A., Godfrey, V. & Koller, B.H. (1999). Growth retardation, DNA repair defects, and lack of spermatogenesis in BRCA1-deficient mice. *Molecular and Cellular Biology*, Vol. 19(10), pp. 7061-7075.

[48] Dacks, J. & Roger, A.J. (1999). The first sexual lineage and the relevance of facultative sex. *Journal of Molecular Evolution*, Vol. 48, pp. 779-783.

[49] Davey, J. (1998). Fusion of a fission yeast. *Yeast*, Vol. 14, pp.1529-1566.

[50] Davidsen, T., Rodland, E.A., Lagesen, K., Seeberg, E., Rognes, T. & Tonjum, T. (2004). Biased distribution of DNA uptake sequences towards genome maintenance genes. *Nucleic Acids Research*, Vol. 32(3), pp. 1050-1058.

[51] De Bont, R., & van Larebeke, N. (2004). Endogenous DNA damage in humans: a review of quantitative data. Mutagenesis, Vol. 19(3), pp.169-185.

[52] Demaneche, S., Kay, E., Gourbiere, F. & Simonet, P. (2001). Natural transformation of *Pseudomonas fluorescens* and *Agrobacterium tumefaciens* in soil. *Applied and Environmental Microbiology*, Vol. 67(6), pp. 2617-2621.

[53] Deng, Z.Y., & Wang, T. (2007). *OsDMC1* is required for homologous pairing in *Oryza sativa. Plant Molecular Biology*, Vol. 65, 31-42.

[54] Dorer, M.S., Fero, J. & Salama, N.R. (2010). DNA damage triggers genetic exchange in *Helicobacter pylori. PloS Pathogens*, Vol. 6(7), pp. 1-10. e1001026

[55] Dubnau, D., Davidoff-Abelson, R., Scher, B. & Cirigliano, C. (1973). Fate of transforming deoxyribonucleic acid after uptake by competent Bacillus subtilis: phenotypic characterization of radiation-sensitive recombination-deficient mutants. Journal of Bacteriology, Vol. 114(1), pp. 273-286.

[56] Edelmann, W., Cohen, P.E., Kneitz, B., Winand, N., Lia, M., Heyer, J., Kolodner, R., Pollard, J.W. & Kucherlapati, R. (1999). Mammalian mutS homologue 5 is required for chromosome pairing in meiosis. Nature Genetics, Vol. 21, pp. 123-127.

[57] Elliott, A.M. & Hayes, R.E. (1953). Mating types in tetrahymena. Biological Bulletin, Vol. 105, pp. 269-284.

[58] Engelmoer, D.J.P. & Rozen, D.E. (2011). Competence increases survival during stress in Streptococcus pneumoniae. Evolution, Vol. 65-12, pp. 3475-3485.

[59] Fisher, H.M. & Aitken, R.J. (1997). Comparative analysis of the ability of precursor germ cells and epididymal spermatozoa to generate reactive oxygen metabolites. The Journal of Experimental Zoology, Vol. 277, pp. 390-400.

[60] Foti, J. J., Devadoss, B., Winkler, J.A., Collins, J.J. & Walker, G.C. (2012). Oxidation of the guanine nucleotide pool underlies cell death by bactericidal antibiotics. Science, Vol. 336, pp. 315-319.

[61] Fraga, C.G., Shigenaga, M.K., Park, J.W., Degan, P. & Ames, B.N. (1990). Oxidative damage to DNA during aging: 8-hydroxy-2'-deoxyguanosine in rat organ DNA and urine. Proceedings of the National Academy of Sciences USA, Vol. 87(12), pp. 4533-4537.

[62] Frols, S., Ajon, M., Wagner, M., Teichmann, D., Zolghadr, B., Folea, M., Boekema, E.J., Driessen, A.J.M., Schleper, C. & Albers, S-V. (2008). UV-inducible cellular aggregation of the hyperthermophilic archaeon *Sulfolobus solfataricus* is mediated by pili formation. *Molecular Microbiology*, Vol. 70(4), pp. 938-952.

[63] Frols, S., White, M.F. & Schleper, C. (2009). Reactions to UV damage in the model archaeon *Sulfolobus solfataricus*. *Biochemical Society Transactions*, Vol. 37(1), 36-41.

[64] Gabaldon, T. & Huynen, M.A. (2003). Reconstruction of the proto-mitochondrial metabolism. *Science*, Vol. 301, p. 609.

[65] Galetzka, D., Weis, E., Kohlschmidt, N., Bitz, O., Stein, R. & Haaf, T. (2007). Expression of somatic DNA repair genes in human testes. *Journal of Cellular Biochemistry*, Vol. 100, pp. 1232-1239.

[66] Game, J.C., Zamb, T.J., Braun, R.J., Resnick, M. and Roth, R.M. (1980). The role of radiation (*rad*) genes in meiotic recombination in yeast. *Genetics*, Vol. 94, pp. 51-68.

[67] Gilley, D. & Blackburn, E.H. (1994). Lack of telemere shortening during senescence in *Paramecium*. *Proceedings of the National Academy of Sciences USA*, Vol. 91, 1955-1958.

[68] Goodgal, S.H. & Herriott, R.M. (1961). Studies on transformations of *Hemophilus influenzae*. I. Competence. *Journal of General Physiology*, Vol. 44, pp. 1201-1227.

[69] Gorelick, R. & Heng, H.H.Q. (2011). Sex reduces genetic variation: A multidisciplinary review. *Evolution*, Vol. 65(4), pp. 1088-1098.

[70] Gray, M.W., Burger, G. & Lang, B.F. (1999). Mitochondrial evolution. *Science* Vol. 283, pp. 1476-1481.

[71] Gross, J. & Bhattacharya, D. (2010). Uniting sex and eukaryote origins in an emerging oxygenic world. *Biology Direct*, Vol. 5:53, pp. 1-20.

[72] Haber, J.E. (1999). DNA recombination: the replication connection. Trends Biochem Sci Vol. 24(7), pp. 271-275.

[73] Halary, S., Malik, S.-B., Lildhar, L., Slarnovits, C.H., Hijri, M., & Corradi, N. (2011). Conserved meiotic machinery in *Glomus* spp., a putatively ancient asexual fungal lineage. *Genome Biology and Evolution*, Vol. 3, pp. 950-958.

[74] Haynes, R.H. (1988). Biological context of DNA repair. In: Friedberg, E.C. & Hanawalt, P.C., editor, Mechanisms and Consequences of DNA Damage Processing, New York, Alan R. Liss, pp. 577-584.

[75] Haynes, R.H. & Kunz, B.A. (1981). DNA repair and mutagenesis in yeast. In: Strathern, J; Jones, E; Broach, J, editors. The Molecular Biology of the Yeast Saccharomyces. Life Cycle and Inheritance. Cold Spring Harbor, N.Y., Cold Spring Harbor Laboratory, 371-414.

[76] Helbock, H.J., Beckman, K.B., Shigenaga, M.K., Walter, P.B., Woodall, A.A., Yeo, H.C. & Ames, B.N. (1998). DNA oxidation matters: the HPLC-electrochemical detection assay of 8-oxo-deoxyguanosine and 8-oxo-guanine. Proceedings of the National Academy of Sciences USA, Vol. 95(1), pp. 288-293.

[77] Henriques, J.A.P. & Moustacchi, E. (1980). Sensitivity to photoaddition of mono- and bifunctional furocoumarins of X-ray sensitive mutants of Saccharomyces cerevisiae. Photochemistry and Photobiology, Vol. 31, pp. 557-563.

[78] Herskowitz, I. (1988). Life cycle of the budding yeast Saccharomyces cerevisiae. Microbiological Reviews, Vol. 52(4), pp. 536- 553.

[79] Hoeijmakers, J.H.J. (2009). DNA damage, aging, and cancer. New England Journal of Medicine, Vol. 361(15), pp. 1475-1485.

[80] Holmes, G.E. & Holmes, N.R. (1986). Accumulation of DNA damages in aging Paramecium tetraurelia. Molecular and General Genetics, Vol. 204, pp. 108-114.

[81] Holthausen, J.T., Wyman, C. & Kanaar, R. (2010). Regulation of DNA strand exchange in homologous recombination. DNA Repair (Amst), Vol. 9(12), pp.1264-1272.

[82] Horandl, E. (2009). A combinational theory for maintenance of sex. *Heredity*, Vol. 103, pp. 445-457.

[83] Hsia, K.T., Millar, M.R., King, S., Selfridge, J., Redhead, N.J., Melton, D.W. & Saunders, P.T.K. (2003). DNA repair gene *Ercc1* is essential for normal spermatogenesis and oogenesis and for functional integrity of germ cell DNA in the mouse. *Development* Vol. 130, pp. 369-378.

[84] Javaux, E.J., Knoll, A.H. & Walter, M.R. (2001). Morphological and ecological complexity in early eukaryote ecosystems. *Nature*, Vol. 412, pp. 66-69.

[85] Ji, G., Long, Y., Zhou, Y., Huang, C., Gu, A. & Wang, X. (2012). Common variants in mismatch repair genes associated with increased risk of sperm DNA damage and male infertility. *BMC Medicine*, 10(49), pp. 1-10.

[86] Johnsborg, O., Eldholm, V. & Håvarstein, L.S. (2007). Natural genetic transformation: prevalence, mechanisms and function. *Research in Microbiology*, Vol. 158(10), pp. 767-778.

[87] Johnson, A. (2003). The biology of mating in *Candida albicans*. *Nature Reviews/Microbiology*, Vol. 1, pp. 106-116.

[88] Joyce, E.F., Tanneti, S.N. & McKim, K.S. (2009). Drosophila Hold'em is required for a subset of meiotic crossovers and interacts with the DNA repair endonuclease complex subunits MEI-9 and ERCC1. *Genetics*, Vol. 181, pp. 335-340.

[89] Kathe, S.D., Shen, G.P. & Wallace, S.S. (2004). Single-stranded breaks in DNA but not oxidative DNA base damages block transcriptional elongation by RNA polymerase II in HeLa cell nuclear extracts. Journal of Biological Chemistry, Vol. 279(18), pp. 18511-18520.

[90] Kelly, S.L., Merrill, C. & Parry, J.M. (1983). Cyclic variations in sensitivity to X-irradiation during meiosis in Saccharomyces cerevisiae. Molecular and General Genetics, Vol. 191, pp. 314-318.

[91] Kidane, D. & Graumann, P.L. (2005). Intracellular protein and DNA dynamics in competent Bacillus subtilis cells. Cell, Vol. 122, pp. 73-84.

[92] Kim, J.S. & Rose, A.M. (1987). The effect of gamma radiation on recombination frequency in Caenorhabditis elegans. Genome, Vol. 29, pp. 457-462.

[93] Kirk, D.L. & Kirk, M.M. (1986). Heat shock elicits production of sexual inducer in Volvox. Science, Vol. 231(4733), pp. 51-54.

[94] Klovstad, M., Abdu, U. & Schupbach, T. (2008). Drosophila brca2 is required for mitotic and meiotic DNA repair and efficient activation of the meiotic recombination checkpoint. PloS Genetics, 4(2): e31.doi:10.1371/journal.pgen.0040031.

[95] Koppen, G. & Verschaeve, L. (2001). The alkaline single-cell gel electrophoresis/ comet assay: a way to study DNA repair in radicle cells of germinating Vicia faba. Folia Biol. (Praha), Vol. 47(2), pp. 50-54.

[96] Kou, Y., Chang, Y., Li, X., Xiao, J. & Wang, S. (2012). The rice *RAD51C* gene is required for the meiosis of both female and male gametocytes and the DNA repair of somatic cells. *Journal of Experimental Botany*, Vol. 63(14), pp. 5323-5335.

[97] Lahr, D.J.G., Parfrey, L.W., Mitchell, E.A.D., Katz, L.A. & Lara, E. (2011). The chastity of amoebae: re-evaluating evidence for sex in amoeboid organisms. *Proceedings of the Royal Society B: Biological Sciences*. Published online 23 March 2011. doi:10.1098/rspb. 2011.0289

[98] Lewis, S.E.M. & Aitken, R.J. (2005). DNA damage to spermatozoa has impacts on fertilization and pregnancy. *Cell Tissue Research*, Vol. 322, pp. 33-41.

[99] Li, J., Harper, L.C., Golubovskaya, I., Wang, C.R., Weber, D., Meeley, R.B., McElver, J., Bowen, B., Cande, W.Z. & Schnable, P.S. (2007). Functional analysis of maize RAD51 in meiosis and double-strand break repair. *Genetics*, Vol. 176, pp. 1469-1482.

[100] Li, W., Chen, C., Markmann-Mulisch, U., Timofejeva, L., Schmeizer, E., Ma, H. & Reiss, B. (2004). The *Arabidopsis AtRAD51* gene is dispensable for vegetative development but required for meiosis. *Proceedings of the National Academy of Sciences USA*, Vol. 101(29), pp. 10596-10601.

[101] Lin, Z. Kong, H., Nei, M. & Ma, H. (2006). Origins and evolution of the *RecA/RAD51* gene family: Evidence for ancient gene duplication and endosymbiotic gene transfer. *Proceedings of the National Academy of Sciences USA*, Vol. 103(27), pp. 10328-10333.

[102] Makker, K., Agarwal, A. & Sharma, R. (2009). Oxidative stress & male infertility. *Indian Journal of Medical Research*, Vol. 129, pp. 357-367.

[103] Malik, S-B., Pightling, A.W., Stefaniak, L.M., Schurko, A.M. & Logsdon, J.M. Jr. (2008). An expanded inventory of conserved meiotic genes provides evidence for sex in *Trichomonas vaginalis*. *Plos One*, Vol. 3(8): e2879. doi:10.1371/journal.pone.0002879.

[104] Malone, R.E. & Esposito, R.E. (1980). The *RAD52* gene is required for homothallic interconversion of mating types and spontaneous mitotic recombination in yeast. *Proceedings of the National Academy of Sciences USA,* Vol. 77(1), pp. 503-507.

[105] Mandon-Pepin, B., Touraine, P., Kuttenn, F., Derbois, C., Rouxel, A., Matsuda, F., Nicolas, A., Cotinot, C. & Fellous, M. (2008). Genetic investigation of four meiotic genes in women with premature ovarian failure. *European Journal of Endocrinology,* Vol. 158, pp. 107-115.

[106] Martin, B., Ruellan, J.M., Angulo, J.F., Devoret, R., and Claverys, J.P. (1992). Identification of the *recA* gene of *Streptococcus pneumoniae*. *Nucleic Acids Research,* Vol. 20(23), p. 6412.

[107] Mechali, M. (2010). Eukaryotic DNA replication origins: many choices for appropriate answers. *Nature Reviews: Molecular Cell Biology,* Vol. 11, pp. 728-738.

[108] Michod, R.E., Wojciechowski, M.F. & Hoelzer, M.A. (1988). DNA repair and the evolution of transformation in the bacterium *Bacillus subtilis*. *Genetics,* Vol. 118(1), pp. 31-39.

[109] Michod, R.E., Bernstein, H. & Nedelcu, A.M. (2008). Adaptive value of sex in microbial pathogens. *Infection, Genetics and Evolution,* Vol. 8(3), pp. 267-285.

[110] Mortier-Barriere, I., de Saizieu, A., Claverys, J.P. & Martin, B. (1998). Competence-specific induction of *recA* is required for full recombination proficiency during transformation in *Streptococcus pneumoniae*. *Molecular Microbiology,* Vol. 27(1), pp. 159-170.

[111] Moynahan, M.E. & Jasin, M. (2010). Mitotic homologous recombination maintains genomic stability and suppresses tumorigenesis. *Nature Reviews/ Molecular Cell Biology,* Vol. 11, pp. 196-207.

[112] Muller, M. & Martin, W. (1999). The genome of *Rickettsia prowazekii* and some thoughts on the origin of mitochondria and hyrogenosomes. *BioEssays,* Vol. 21, pp. 377-381.

[113] Murayama, Y., Kurokawa, Y., Mayanagi, K. & Iwasaki, H. (2008). Formation and branch migration of Holliday junctions mediated by eukaryotic recombinases. Nature, Vol. 451(7181), pp. 1018-1021.

[114] Nakamura, J., Walker, V.E., Upton, P.B., Chiang, S.Y., Kow, Y.W. & Swenberg, J.A. (1998). Highly sensitive apurinic/apyrimidinic site assay can detect spontaneous and chemically induced depurination under physiological conditions. Cancer Research, Vol. 58(2), pp. 222-225.

[115] Nedelcu, A.M. & Michod, R.E. (2003). Sex as a response to oxidative stress: The effect of antioxidants on sexual induction in a facultatively sexual lineage. Proceedings of the Royal Society London B (suppl.) Vol. 270, pp. S136-S139.

[116] Nedelcu, A.M., Marcu, O. & Michod, R.E. (2004). Sex as a response to oxidative stress: a two-fold increase in cellular reactive oxygen species activates sex genes. Proceedings of the Royal Society London B, Vol. 271, pp. 1591-1596.

[117] Nili, H.A., Mozdarani, H. & Pellestor, F. (2011). Impact of DNA damage on the frequency of sperm chromosomal aneuploidy in normal and subfertile men. Iranian Biomedical Journal, 15(4), 122-129.

[118] O'Connor, M., Wopat, A. & Hanson, R.S. (1977). Genetic transformation in *Methylobacterium organophilum*. *Journal of General Microbiology*, Vol. 98, pp.265-272.

[119] Oktay, K., Kim, J. Y. Barad, D. & Babayev, S.N. (2010). Association of *BRCA1* mutations with occult primary ovarian insufficiency: A possible explanation for the link between infertility and breast/ovarian cancer risks. *Journal of Clinical Oncology*, Vol 28(2), pp. 240-244.

[120] Patel, G.B., Nash, J.H.E., Agnew, B.J. & Sprott, G.D. (1994). Natural and electroporation-mediated transformation of *Methanococcus voltae* protoplasts. *Applied and Environmental Microbiology*, Vol. 60(3), pp. 903-907.

[121] Paul, C., Murray, A.A., Spears, N. & Saunders, P.T. (2008). A single, mild, transient scrotal heat stress causes DNA damage, subfertility and impairs formation of blastocysts in mice. *Reproduction*, Vol. 136(1), pp. 73-84.

[122] Pittman, D.L., Cobb, J., Schimenti, K.J., Wilson, L.A., Cooper, D.M., Brignull, E., Handel, M.A. & Schimenti, J.C. (1998). Meiotic prophase arrest with failure of chromosome synapsis in mice deficient for *Dmc1*, a germline-specific *RecA* homolog. *Molecular Cell*, Vol. 1, pp. 697-705.

[123] Preston, C.R., Flores, C. & Engels, W.R. (2006). Age-dependent usage of double-strand-break repair pathways. *Current Biology*, Vol. 16, pp. 2009-2015.

[124] Prudhommeau, C. & Proust, J. (1973). UV irradiation of polar cells of *Drosophila melanogaster* embryos. V. A study of the meiotic recombination in females with chromosomes of different structure. *Mutation Research*, Vol. 22, pp. 63-66.

[125] Raina, J.L. & Modi, V.V. (1972). Deoxyribonucleate binding and transformation in *Rhizobium japonicum*. *Journal of Bacteriology*, Vol. 111(2), pp. 356-360.

[126] Ramesh, M.A., Malik, S.B. & Logsdon, J.M. (2005). A phylogenomic inventory of meiotic genes: Evidence for sex in *Giardia* and an early eukaryotic origin of meiosis. *Current Biology*, Vol. 15, pp. 185-191.

[127] Rasmusen, A. (1984). Effects of DNA-repair-deficient mutants on somatic and germ line mutagenesis in the UZ system of *Drosophila melanogaster*. *Mutation Research*, Vol. 141, pp. 29-33.

[128] Reeves, R.J. & Jackson, R.M. (1974). Stimulation of sexual reproduction in *Phytophthora* by damage. *Journal of General Microbiology*, Vol. 84, pp. 303-310.

[129] Roberts, C.J. & Lowe, C.R. (1975). Where have all the conceptions gone? *Lancet*, Vol. 305(7905), pp. 498-499.

[130] Rosenshine, I., Tchelet, R. & Mevarech, M. (1989). The mechanism of DNA transfer in the mating system of an archaebacterium. *Science*, Vol. 245(4924), pp. 1387-1389.

[131] Ruderfer, D.M., Pratt, S.C., Seidel, H.S. & Kruglyak, L. (2006). Population genomic analysis of outcrossing and recombination in yeast. *Nature Genetics*, Vol. 38(9), 1077-1081.

[132] Sagan, C. (1973). Ultraviolet selection pressure on the earliest organisms. *Journal of Theoretical Biology*, Vol. 39, pp. 195-200.

[133] Sager, R. & Granick, S. (1954). Nutritional control of sexuality in *Chlamydomonas reinhardi*. *Journal of General Physiology*, Vol. 37, pp.729-742.

[134] Saito, Y., Taguchi, H. & Akamatsu, T. (2006). Fate of transforming bacterial genome following incorporation into competent cells of *Bacillus subtilis*: a continuous length of incorporated DNA. *Journal of Bioscience and Bioengineering*, Vol. 101(3), pp. 257-262.

[135] Sakai, A., Nakanishi, M., Yoshiyama, K. & Maki, H. (2006). Impact of reactive oxygen species on spontaneous mutagenesis in *Escherichia coli*. *Genes to Cells*, Vol. 11, pp. 767-778.

[136] Sakano, K., Oikawa, S., Hasegawa, K & Kawanishi, S. (2001). Hydroxyurea induces site-specific DNA damage via formation of hydrogen peroxide and nitric oxide. *Japanese Journal of Cancer*, Vol. 92(11), pp. 1166-1174.

[137] Sandler, S.J., Satin, L.H., Samra, H.S. & Clark, A.J. (1996). *recA*-like genes from three archaean species with putative protein products similar to Rad51 and Dmc1 proteins of the yeast *Saccharomyces cerevisiae*. *Nucleic Acids Research*, Vol. 24(11), 2125-2132.

[138] San Filippo, J., Sung, P. & Klein, H. (2008). Mechanism of eukaryotic homologous recombination. *Annual Review of Biochemistry*, Vol. 77, pp. 229-257.

[139] Sauvageau, S., Stasiak, A.Z., Banville, I., Ploquin, M. Stasiak, A. & Masson, J.Y. (2005). Fission yeast Rad51 and Dmc1, two efficient DNA recombinases forming helical nucleoprotein filaments. *Molecular and Cellular Biology*, Vol. 25(11), pp. 4377-4387.

[140] Schewe, M.J., Suzuki, D.T. & Erasmus, U. (1971). The genetic effects of mitomycin C in *Drosophila melanogaster*. II. Induced meiotic recombination. *Mutation Research*, Vol. 12, pp. 269-279.

[141] Sehorn, M.G., Sigurdsson, S., Bussen, W., Unger, V.M. & Sung, P. (2004). Human meiotic recombinase Dmc1 promotes ATP-dependent homologous DNA strand exchange. *Nature*, Vol. 429, pp. 433-437.

[142] Shinohara, A., Ogawa, H., Matsuda, Y., Ushio, N., Ikeo, K. & Ogawa, T. (1993). Cloning of human, mouse and fission yeast recombination genes homologous to *RAD51* and *recA*. *Nature Genetics*, Vol. 4, pp. 239-243.

[143] Slupphaug, G., Kavli, B. & Krokan, H.E. (2003). The interacting pathways for prevention and repair of oxidative DNA damage. *Mutation Research*, Vol. 531, pp. 231-251.

[144] Smith-Sonneborn, J. (1979). DNA repair and longevity assurance in *Paramecium tetraurelia*. *Science*, Vol. 203, pp. 1115 – 1117.

[145] Soleimani, R., Heytens, E., Darzynkiewicz, Z. & Oktay, K. (2011). Mechanisms of chemotherapy-induced human ovarian aging: double strand DNA breaks and microvascular compromise. *Aging*, Vol. 3(8), pp. 1-12.

[146] Solomon, J.M. & Grossman, A.D. (1996). Who's competent and when: regulation of natural genetic competence in bacteria. *Trends in Genetics*, Vol. 12(4), pp.150-155.

[147] Staeva-Vieira, E., Yoo, S. & Lehmann, R. (2003). An essential role of DmRad51/SpnA in DNA repair and meiotic checkpoint control. The EMBO Journal, Vol. 22(21), pp. 5863-5874.

[148] Stohl, E.A., Gruenig, M.C., Cox, M.M. & Seifert, H.S. (2011). Purification and characterization of the RecA protein from Neisseria gonorrhoeae. PloS ONE, 6(2), e17101.

[149] Stohl, E.A. & Seifert, H.S. (2006). Neisseria gonorrhoeae DNA recombination and repair enzymes protect against oxidative damage caused by hydrogen peroxide. Journal of Bacteriology, Vol. 188(21), pp. 7645-7651.

[150] Story, R.M., Bishop, D.K., Kleckner, N. & Steitz, T.A. (1993). Structural relationship of bacterial RecA proteins to recombination proteins from bacteriophage T4 and yeast. Science, Vol. 259(5103), pp. 1892 – 1896.

[151] Suzuki, D.T. & Parry, D.M. (1964). Crossing over near the centromere of chromosome 3 in Drosophila melanogaster females. Genetics, Vol. 50, pp. 1427-1432.

[152] Takanami, T., Mori, A., Takahashi, H. & Higashitani, A. (2000). Hyper-resistance of meiotic cells to radiation due to a strong expression of a single RecA-like gene in Caenorhabditis elegans. Nucleic Acids Research, Vol. 28(21), pp. 4232-4236.

[153] Takanami, T., Zhang, Y., Aoki, H., Abe, T., Yoshida, S., Takahashi, H., Horiuchi, S. & Higashitani, A. (2003). Efficient repair of DNA damage induced by heavy ion particles in meiotic prophase I nuclei of Caenorhabditis elegans. Journal of Radiation Research, Vol. 44, pp. 271-276.

[154] Terasawa, M., Shinohara, A., Hotta, Y., Ogawa, H. & Ogawa, T. (1995). Localization of RecA-like recombination proteins on chromosomes of the lily at various meiotic stages. Genes and Development, Vol. 9, pp. 925-934.

[155] Tice, R.R. & Setlow, R.B. (1985). DNA repair and replication in aging organisms and cells. In: Finch, E.E. & Schneider, E.L. (eds.) Handbook of the Biology of Aging. Van Nostrand Reinhold, New York. pp. 173-224.

[156] Tichy, E.D., Pillai, R., Deng, L., Liang, L., Tischfield, J., Schwemberger, S.J., Babcock, G.F. & Stambrook, P.J. (2010). Mouse embryonic stem cells, but not somatic cells, pre-

dominantly use homologous recombination to repair double-strand breaks. Stem Cells and Development, Vol. 19(11), pp. 1699-1711.

[157] Titus, S., Li, F., Stobezki, R., Akula, K., Unsal, E., Jeong, K., Dickler, M., Robson, M., Moy, F., Goswami, S. & Oktay, K. (2013). Impairment of BRCA1-related DNA double-strand break repair leads to ovarian aging in mice and humans. Science Translational Medicine, Vol. 5(172ra21), pp. 1-12.

[158] Unal, E., Kinde, B. & Amon, A. (2011). Gametogenesis eliminates age-induced cellular damage and resets life span in yeast. Science, Vol. 332, pp. 1554-1557.

[159] Vilenchik, M.M. & Knudson, A.G. (2003). Endogenous DNA double-strand breaks: production, fidelity of repair, and induction of cancer. Proceedings of the National Academy of Sciences USA, Vol. 100(22), pp. 12871-12876.

[160] Washburn, R.S. & Gottesman, M.E. (2011). Transcription termination maintains chromosome integrity. *Proceedings of the National Academy of Sciences USA*, Vol. 108(2), pp. 792-797.

[161] Wei, K., Kucherlapati, R. & Edelmann, W. (2002). Mouse models for human DNA mismatch-repair gene defects. *TRENDS in Molecular Medicine*, Vol. 8(7), pp. 346-353.

[162] Wilcox, A.J., Weinberg, C.R., O'Connor, J.F., Baird, D.D., Schlatterer, J.P., Canfield, R.E., Armstrong, E.G. & Nisula, B.C. (1988). Incidence of early loss of pregnancy. *New England Journal of Medicine*, Vol. 319(4), pp. 189-194.

[163] Wood, E.R., Ghane, F. & Grogan, D.W. (1997). Genetic responses to the thermophilic archaeon *Sulfolobus acidocaldarius* to short-wavelength UV light. *Journal of Bacteriology*, Vol. 179(18), pp. 5693-5698.

[164] Worrell, V.E., Nagle, D.P., McCarthy, D. & Eisenbraun, A. (1988). Genetic transformation system in the archaebacterium *Methanobacterium thermoautotrophicum* Marburg. *Journal of Bacteriology*, Vol. 170(2), pp. 653-656.

[165] Yoshida, K., Kondoh, G., Matsuda, Y., Habu, T., Nishimune, Y. & Morita, T. (1998). The mouse *recA*-like gene *dmc1* is required for homologous chromosome synapsis during meiosis. *Molecular Cell*, Vol. 1, pp. 707-718.

[166] Zeyl, C.W. & Otto, S.P. (2007). A short history of recombination in yeast. *Trends in Ecology and Evolution*, Vol. 22(5), pp. 223-225.

Chapter 4

Meiosis: Its Origin According to the Viral Eukaryogenesis Theory

Philip Bell

Additional information is available at the end of the chapter

http://dx.doi.org/10.5772/56876

1. Introduction

The core meiotic machinery is largely universal in eukaryotes indicating that a substantial proportion of the meiotic machinery had already evolved in early eukaryotes [1]. Since there appear to be no close homologues to meiosis and the sexual cycle in either the bacterial or archaeal domains, it seems reasonable to propose that the origin of meiosis appears to be associated with the early origin of the eukaryotes themselves. Given the complexity and the level of integration of the intricate processes required to effectively maintain meiosis and a sexual cycle, it has been difficult to envisage how the full meiotic and sexual cycles could appear in the eukaryotic domain, without clear homologues in the prokaryotic domains of life. This is a particular challenge if all life descends directly from a Last Universal Common Ancestor (the LUCA hypothesis) and life evolves only according to the classical neo-Darwinian principles of incremental changes. It is not surprising then that the origin of sex, (and by extension the origin of meiosis), has been described as the queen of evolutionary problems [2].

If we investigate the characteristic features of the eukaryotic domain, we find that meiosis is only one of a wide array of features that have such a wide distribution within the eukaryotes that they appear to have been present and almost fully developed in the ancestor of all living eukaryotes [3]. These features include the nucleus, endomembrane systems, linear chromosomes with telomeres, mitochondria, peroxisomes, the cell division apparatus, mitosis, nuclear pores, mRNA capping, introns, the spliceosomal apparatus and the nuclear pore proteins [3]. Given this range of complex inter-related characters apparently present at the origin of the eukaryotes, the earliest common eukaryotic ancestor was clearly very different in design compared to any cells of the bacterial or archaeal domains. In addition, it has been clear for some time that the eukaryotic genome is an ancient chimera, a blend between bacterial metabolic genes and archaeal information processing genes [4]. Together, these observations make the evolutionary relationship between the eukaryotes and the prokaryotes very challenging to elucidate since there is apparently an insurmountable chasm between eukaryotic and prokaryotic cells.

If we accept the paradigm of a 'Last Universal Common Ancestor' (e.g. LUCA), the apparently abrupt emergence of the eukaryotes in their modern form without transitional organisms is a major challenge to the classic Darwinian view of evolution. In particular, if we restrict our understanding of evolution to that of the classical neo-Darwinian school of evolution, every small evolutionary step leading to the origin of the first eukaryote should have conferred a selective advantage on the cell, thus the evolution of the complex traits observed in the transition from prokaryotes to eukaryotes (or visa versa) should have proceeded via small steps, each of which provided a selective advantage during the transition in cellular design. However, the transition in design between prokaryotic and eukaryotic design involves changes so profound, no convincing series of plausible small changes, each with its own selective advantage has been proposed that would begin to allow for this transition. In addition, no such transitional forms have been recognised either as fossils or survived as 'missing links'. Simply put, there are no credible evolutionarily intermediates between the prokaryotic and eukaryotic domains. That is, there are no organisms found with a eukaryote-like nucleus without linear chromosomes, or a mitochondrion without an endoplasmic reticulum, or a meiotic replication cycle without a cytoskeleton, that would indicate a stepwise evolutionary acquisition of critical eukaryotic features. Rather, all eukaryotes that we can observe today appear to descend from a common ancestor that already possessed a complex suite of multiple characteristics and none are descended from any earlier intermediates without many of the critical characteristic eukaryotic features [3].

One possible solution to this evolutionary impasse lies in the symbiogenic mode of evolution. A major role for symbiogenesis in evolution was postulated over 100 years ago when it was proposed that chloroplasts were descended from free living photosynthetic organisms [5]. However, for reasons that are difficult to decipher [6], the theory was scorned by the scientific community. By the early 1960's the theory drew attention in some textbooks only as a 'bad penny that has been in circulation far too long' [7]. It took a re-launch of the theory by scientists such as Lynn Margulis in the late 1960's and 1970's [8] to resurrect symbiogenesis as a mainstream scientific topic and combat the resistance to the concept. Despite the scientific community's dogmatic reluctance to embrace the symbiogenic model for evolution, it is now the accepted paradigm for the evolution of key eukaryotic features such as both the chloroplasts and mitochondria [9].

The symbiogenic mode of evolution can be interpreted as a specialised form of neo-Darwinian evolution, since it involves the gradual evolution of two organisms that obtain some mutual advantage from their relationship (mutualism) such that the evolutionary trajectories of each organism are related to each other. In the symbiogenic mode of evolution, each of the organisms are subject to classical neo-Darwinian selection where small infinitesimal changes in their individual genetic codes allow for closer and closer integration with the other member so that each organism evolves to adapt to the presence of the other. In some cases the intimate relationship between the two organisms effectively creates a third organism that is unlike either ancestor alone. A classic example is that of lichens, which are composed of a photobiont (cyanobacteria or alga) and a fungal host that have co-evolved to such an extent they are classified as "lichen" species, despite the fact that each lichen consists of at least two separate organisms that can relatively easily enter into and leave the symbiotic relationship [10]. Lichens demonstrate how a symbiogenic mode of evolution can allow for complex changes in organismal design to appear whilst adhering strictly to the neo-Darwinian mode of gradualistic evolution for each of the organisms involved.

A case of symbiogenesis directly relevant to the origin of the eukaryotes is the case of the evolution of the chloroplast. As mentioned above, the idea that the eukaryotic chloroplast is symbiotic in origin is an old one [5] and despite being dogmatically resisted by the scientific community for over 50 years it is currently supported by so many lines of evidence that it is a widely considered incontrovertible [11]. Critically the presence of symbiogenic chloroplasts provides a clue as to the timing of the eukaryotic divergences and thus addresses one of the critical issues of the origin of the eukaryotes. In the case of chloroplasts, it is clear that they originally derive from a prokaryotic cyanobacteria of domain bacteria [12]. Since the chloroplast could not have originated prior to the origin of the cyanobacteria, it is clear that the eukaryotic plant lineage as a whole could not have evolved prior to the evolution and differentiation of the cyanobacteria from other bacterial groups. Therefore the first eukaryotic plant cell (presumably an alga) could not have evolved before photosynthesis had evolved in the bacterial domain, and the cyanobacteria had diverged from the other bacteria both photosynthetic and non photosynthetic. With regards to the timing of the origin of the ancestor of all modern eukaryotes, chloroplasts are not one of the universal eukaryotic features, as they are only found in the photosynthetic lineages, and thus the symbiogenic origin of the chloroplast does not inform us about the origin of the eukaryotes themselves since it seems likely that plant cell ancestors were eukaryotic before they entered into the symbiosis with the cyanobacteria. However the endosymbiotic origin of the chloroplasts is an important example since it clearly shows that symbiogenesis can and has made a major contribution to the evolution of at least some complex features of modern eukaryotes.

If we examine mitochondria rather than the chloroplasts, we find that they are also derived from a symbiogenic origin [9], but unlike the chloroplasts, mitochondria are one of the unique universal eukaryotic features that appeared prior to the origin of the last universal ancestor of the eukaryotes alive today [3]. Thus, like the transition from circular to linear chromosomes, or the acquisition of a nucleus, or the invention of mRNA capping, the origin of the mitochondria is associated with the origin of the last eukaryotic common ancestor. This is highly informative since if the mitochondrion is descended from a bacterial endosymbiont, and the last universal ancestor of the eukaryotes possessed a mitochondrion, then the last universal ancestor of the living eukaryotes could only have originated after the origin of the bacterial domain. According to this logic, the existence of mitochondria in the last eukaryotic common ancestor implies not only that the eukaryotes emerged after the bacterial domain had originated, but also that the eukaryotes evolved in a world that already possessed bacteria. Phylogenetic analysis of the mitochondria shows that they are not just descended from a generic ancestral bacterium, but rather they descend from an alpha-proteobacteria probably related to the Ricksettsiales [13], and thus the last ancestor of all modern eukaryotes must have evolved after the bacterial domain had already differentiated into a wide range of bacterial phyla, including the extensive proteobacterial divisions.

If the mitochondria shares a common ancestor specifically with alpha-proteobacteria, then the ancestor of all modern eukaryotes must have emerged from an environment in which the bacteria had already evolved into their modern groups, and therefore presumably their modern forms. This is consistent with other lines of evidence such as the fossil record which suggests that the first traces of eukaryotic cells post dates that of recognisable cyanobacterial fossils by over a billion years [7].

If the bacteria were already essentially modern in design before the evolution of the last eukaryotic common ancestor, the question arises as to what other life forms were present. With regards to the archaea, given that fossil evidence suggests that methanogenesis arose greater than 2.8 billion years ago [14], and methanogenesis is an exclusively archaeal process, it would appear that the archaea were also present prior to the origin of the eukaryotes. This is confirmed by the observation that the ancestral eukaryotic genome is a chimera of bacterial and archaeal genes [4] which indicates that prokaryotes of the archaeal domain were also present at the origin of the eukaryotes. Significantly, recent research confidently indicates that the genome of the last common ancestor of all extant archaea apparently was at least as large and complex as that of typical modern organisms in this domain of cellular life. [15] The evidence thus suggests that both bacteria and archaea were highly evolved and already differentiated into major groups when the eukaryotes evolved and therefore the eukaryotes evolved in a 'prokaryotic world' which contained at least bacteria and archaea.

It also seems likely that viruses, phages, and plasmids were also present in this 'prokaryotic world' as there is evidence that the last common universal ancestor of cellular organisms was infected by a number of different viruses. [16] Further support for the proposal that complex DNA viruses predated the origin of the eukaryotes comes from analysis of some of the most complex known viruses, the NCLDV viruses. Phylogenetic studies on the NCLDV viruses have shown that this class of DNA viruses was present before or at the origin of the last universal eukaryotic ancestor. [17], [18], [19] In addition, phylogenetic analysis of key nuclear/NCLDV signature genes such as mRNA capping enzymes indicate that they branch from the phylogenetic branch leading to the earliest eukaryotes. [20] Further support for the existence of phage/viruses at or close to the origin of the eukaryotes comes from molecular analysis of mitochondria where the enzyme used in transcription of mitochondrial genomes are related to T7 phage RNA polymerases rather than typical bacterial RNA polymerases. [21] The phage version is found in the majority of the groups of eukaryotes, with the only currently known exception being the RNA polymerase in the protist *Reclinomonas*. [21] Since the phage version is almost ubiquitous in eukaryotic mitochondria, it suggests that the T7 bacteriophage were present close to the ancestor of all living eukaryotes.

In conclusion, several lines of evidence can be used to argue with some degree of confidence that the ancestor of all modern eukaryotes descends from an ancestor that appeared relatively 'late' in the evolution of life on earth, and that it lived in a 'prokaryotic world' in which bacteria, archaea and complex DNA viruses had already evolved into recognisably modern forms.

http://dx.doi.org/10.5772/56876

Furthermore, the symbiogenic origin of the mitochondria and the chloroplasts in algal/plant lineages indicates that symbiogensis was a critical evolutionary process active in the origin and early evolution of the eukaryotes. It is in this prokaryotic world in which the Viral Eukaryogenesis theory for the origin of the eukaryotes, meiosis, and the sexual cycle is set.

2. The Viral Eukaryogenesis theory : A prokaryotic community evolves into the eukaryotic cell

At its simplest level, the Viral Eukaryogenesis theory proposes that the eukaryotic cell is descended from a prokaryotic world community consisting of three phylogenetically unrelated organisms. These three organisms were, an archaeal ancestor of the eukaryotic cytoplasm, an alpha-proteobacterial ancestor of the mitochondria and a viral ancestor of the nucleus. [20] Although it is now widely accepted that the eukaryotic mitochondria is descended from an endosymbiotic bacterium, it is the idea that the eukaryotic nucleus could be a viral endosymbiont that is usually considered to be a radical or 'far-fetched' aspect of the Viral Eukaryogenesis theory. It would appear to be particularly radical due to what I believe to be prejudices and outdated paradigms about viruses. For example, viruses were long defined by their small size and inability to replicate outside of a cell, and thus the viruses failed to even meet the definition of life, and were more like inanimate poisons that could be crystallised and stored as an inert substance. Even the name virus is derived from the Latin word for poison which implies both that viruses are entirely destructive of life, and that they are more like a liquid chemical poison than a living organism. In the original version of the Viral Eukaryogenesis theory, [20] it was proposed that eukaryotic nucleus was descended from a pox-like virus (which at the time was one of the most complex viruses known), a scourge of humanity, and not exactly a wholesome image for a relative, no matter how distant.

Over the last decade, however, the established viral paradigm has gradually been modified by the discovery of complex NCLDV viruses such as the Mimivirus, Mamavirus, Megavirus and CroV viruses. These viruses are so large and complex that they exceed the complexity of some living prokaryotes, and some authors have even proposed that the Mimiviruses and its kin are a fourth domain or supergroup of life, rivalling the bacteria, archaea and eukaryotes. [17, 18] The Mimivirus was the first of these giant viruses to be discovered, and its discovery has led to the realisation that viruses can be far more complex than previously thought. [22] Indeed, the Mimivirus was unlikely to have been found using standard methods, because the old viral paradigm included a criteria that they could pass through a Chamberland filter that would filter out bacteria sized particles like the Mimivirus. Sequencing of the Mimvirus and other members of the giant viruses has revealed that not only are the viruses large, they are genetically complex, possessing many features that were previously considered to be restricted to cellular organisms. [22] Amongst the > 1000 genes present in the giant viruses are many genes involved in translation, transcription, and genetic information processing. [22]

One of the objections to the idea that a virus could be the ancestor of the eukaryotic nucleus is that the viruses are non-living and therefore not really a valid candidate to be an endosymbiotic ancestor of the eukaryotic nucleus. However, if one makes a comparison between the modern Mimivirus and the modern bacterium *Rickettsia belli* it can be seen that in terms of size, complexity and habitat there are many similarities between these two organisms despite one being a virus, and the other being a bacterium related to the eukaryotic mitochondrion. In terms of size, these two organisms are fairly similar, and in fact the Mimivirus was named for the fact that it was a 'Mimicking microbe'. In terms of complexity, the organisms are also similar, with both possessing genomes in the range of 1200-1500 protein coding genes, [22, 23] both organisms are membrane bound, and both possess genes involved in translation, transcription and genetic information processing. Most strikingly however, is that both organisms are obligate internal parasites, and both are known to be capable of replicating in the same host. That is, the Mimivirus was originally discovered infecting *Acanthamoeba polyphaga,* [22] a host in which *Rickettsia bellii* can also replicate. [23] Significantly in terms of the Viral Eukaryogenesis theory, phylogenetic analysis of the genes of both these organisms show that they descend from ancestors that existed before the eukaryotes arose. [9, 17, 18, 19, 20] If it can be accepted that an alpha-proteobacterial ancestor of Rickettsia could have established a permanent endosymbiosis within the lineage leading to the origin of the eukaryotes and thus evolved into the mitochondria, there seems no scientific reason why an ancestor of an equally complex obligate internal parasite like the Mimivirus could not have similarly established a permanent endosymbiosis within the lineage leading to the origin of the eukaryotes and thus evolved into the nucleus. Of course, in the Viral Eukaryogenesis theory, it is proposed that one critical difference between the endosymbionts was that during the evolution of the eukaryotes, the alpha-proteobacterial genome was dramatically reduced in complexity as it evolved into the mitochondria whilst the viral genome increased in complexity as it evolved into the nucleus. Presumably this difference in evolutionary trajectory occurred due to the different functions of the organisms within the community as they evolved specialised functions within the eukaryotic cell; the mitochondria as a centre for active metabolism, and the nucleus as a centre for transcription and replication of genetic material.

One consequence of the proposed derivation of the eukaryotes from three members of the 'proto-eukaryotic' community, is that the modern eukaryotic genome should be a palimpsest of genes derived from the three phylogenetic sources. In this way the VE theory provides a basis for understanding the observation that the eukaryotic nucleus is a chimera of genes derived from bacterial and archaeal sources [4] and explains why the information processing genes of eukaryotes are generally of an archaeal nature, whereas genes of more general metabolic nature are of a bacterial origin. As explained in the VE theory, the tripartite consortium initially contained three separate but interacting genomes. The archaeal host genome possessed genes characteristic of those in archaeal organisms, and thus the ribosomes, translation apparatus, DNA metabolism genes, cell replication genes and other general metabolic genes of the cytoplasm would have originally been derived from archaeal origins. In contrast, the viral genome possessed genes characteristic of those of the NCLDV viral lineage, and thus the genes for virus/nuclear replication, assembly, membrane folding, DNA replication, DNA maintenance, and mRNA capping would have originally been derived from viral origins. These viral genes would also be genes that evolved to interact with the archaeal information processing apparatus since the virus was dependent on host archaeal machinery for translation and replication. Finally, the third genome, the bacterial genome, possessed genes characteristic of those in bacterial organisms, and thus the future mitochondrial ribosomes, translation apparatus and many metabolic genes would have originally been derived from bacterial origins. It is proposed that the different functions and thus evolutionary trajectories of the genomes of the three members of the consortium influenced their location in modern eukaryotes. In the case of the original alpha-protoebacterial endosymbiont, despite being separated from the future viral/nuclear genome by the symbiont membrane, the vast majority of genes of the original endosymbiont were either re-located to the viral/nuclear genome or lost, with only a few genes remaining in the modern mitochondrial genome and, in the even more reduced hydrogenosomes, the endosymbiont genome as a separate entity completely disappeared. In the case of the host archaeal genome, it is proposed that its 'ínformation processing' genes, where needed, were re-located to the future viral/nuclear genome, and the archaeal genome as a separate entity, like that of the hydrogenosome genome, completely disappeared. As a result of these processes, the eukaryotes ended up with two independently replicating genomes, the much reduced mitochondrial genome, and the greatly expanded viral/nuclear genome representing a chimera of genes derived from the original virus, the archaeal host and the a range of genes from bacterial endosymbionts including the ancestor of the mitochondria.

As shown in Figure 1, it is proposed that the unique genetic architecture of the eukaryotes arose because the eukaryotic cell is the descendent of a symbiogenic prokaryotic world community rather than a single ancestral cell. It is proposed that the community became integrated to such an extent that, like the lichens, we see the components of the community as a single organism, which we currently recognise as the eukaryotic cell. Thus the unique design of the eukaryotic cell arose because of the integration of the three lineages into a single unit. [20] It is further proposed that the co-ordination of their replication cycles led to the evolution of mitosis, meiosis and the unique eukaryotic cell cycle. [24]

A key aspect of Viral Eukaryogenesis theory that differentiates it from many other models is that it proposes that the eukaryotes did not result from a single chance 'event' such as a chance fusion between cells, but rather that the three symbiogenic lineages that were involved in the emergence of the eukaryotic cell were evolutionarily linked together and the eukaryotic cell we see today resulted from a process that over time increasingly linked each of the organisms together. That is, the archaeal lineage is linked to the evolution of the bacterial lineage because of a mutualistic symbiotic relationship between the two organisms, and the virus and the archaea are evolutionarily linked together in a symbiotic host/parasite relationship. As a result the three lineages were found together in the same ecological community, and they shared a linked evolutionary process that lead to the evolution of the eukaryotic cell. In this community, each member of the consortium evolved according to classical neo-Darwinian models, however as they became more and more integrated, they eventually became unrecognisable as separate organisms, but rather were integrated into a single permanent consortium that we call the eukaryotic cell.

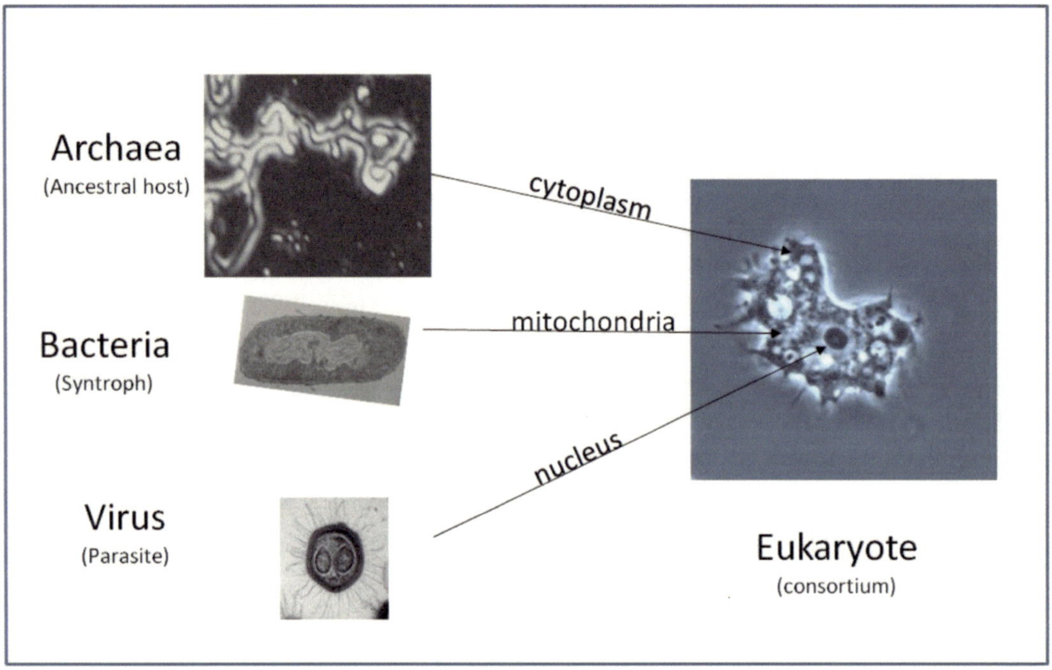

Figure 1. The eukaryotic cell evolves from a prokaryotic world community/consortium. In the Viral Eukaryogenesis theory, the eukaryotic cell is descended from a consortium of three originally independent prokaryotic world organisms. The eukaryotic cytoplasm is descended from an archaeal cell that did not possess a cell wall and was subject to infection by a variety of agents including a range of bacteria and viruses. The eukaryotic mitochondrion is descended from an alpha-proteobacteria that was originally in a syntrophic relationship with the archaeal host, and eventually invaded the host cytoplasm and established an permanent endosymbiotic presence in the host cell. The eukaryotic nucleus is descended from a NCLDV virus that was originally in a parasitic relationship with the archaeal host, and eventually established a permanent lysogenic presence within the host cytoplasm. The three organisms of the consortium eventually shared a common evolutionary trajectory and eventually evolved into the eukaryotic cell. In the process of permanently establishing the 'eukaryotic cell', the viral ancestor of the nucleus took over the roles of DNA replication and transcription by means of its capping/cap binding proteins that directed preferential translation of the viral transcripts into proteins. As a result, the virus became the genetic information processing centre of the cell and gradually acquired genes from the other organisms. The alpha proteobacterial ancestor of the mitochondria transferred the majority of its genes to the virus/nucleus in the process of evolving into the mitochondria, and in the case of hydrogenosomes, all of its genes. The host archaeal cytoplasm maintained its role in translation of mRNA transcripts and eventually transferred all of its 'eukaryotic' genes to the nucleus.

3. An archaeal ancestor of the eukaryotic cytoplasm

An archaea is proposed as the ancestor of the eukaryotic cytoplasm in the Viral Eukaryogenesis theory primarily because it is clear that the eukaryotic ribosomes are more closely related to those of the archaea than the bacteria. [4] More specifically, an archaea without a cell wall is proposed because it can be argued that the eukaryotic ancestor did not possess a cell wall since many modern eukaryotes such as animals do not possess cell walls, and those that do, possess a range of cell wall materials (eg mannoproteins in yeast, cellulose in plants, etc) that were most likely evolved independently of each other. [20] There have been at least two archaea described that do not possess a cell wall, *Thermoplasma* and *Methanoplasma elizabethii.* It has been proposed several times that *Thermoplasma* may have been related to the ancestry of the eukaryotes. [25, 26] However, *Methanoplasma elizabethii* is proposed in the Viral Eukaryogenesis theory as an archetype for the ancestor of the eukaryotic cytoplasm. *M. elizabethii* is a modern member of a syntrophic consortium consisting of bacteria and archaea that metabolise fatty acids into methane. [27] Although, '*M. elizabethii*', is not expected to be particularly closely related to the ancestor of the eukaryotic cytoplasm, it was chosen because it is illustrative of the evolutionary forces that could link the evolution of an archaeal ancestor of the cytoplasm with a bacterial ancestor of the mitochondrion. In the modern consortium in which *M. elizabethii* is found, the bacteria break down fatty acids and produce hydrogen and carbon dioxide as waste products, which are used by the archaeon as a source of raw materials for methanogenesis. [27] This type of syntrophic relationship provides an evolutionary and ecological linkage between the two species. In the Viral Eukaryogenesis theory it is proposed that a syntrophic relationship between an archaeon and a bacterium ensured the long-term co-evolution of the two species since they existed in a mutually advantageous relationship. Although not fully elucidated, the recent discovery of anaerobic methane oxidation consortia has demonstrated that syntrophy between methane oxidising archaea (ANME) and bacteria occurs on a global scale and is responsible for major geochemical carbon cycles in the earth's biosphere. [28] Critically the ANME type syntrophy is independent of the presence of oxygen and these types of syntrophy could have been abundant prior to the time that the first eukaryotes appeared.

4. A bacterial ancestor of the mitochondrion

An alpha-proteobacteria is chosen in the Viral Eukaryogenesis theory to be the ancestor of the mitochondria since it is clear from phylogenetic and structural studies that the mitochondria are descended from an alpha-proteobacterium. [29] For example, the genes of the electron transport chain in the mitochondria are clearly homologous and specifically related to those of the alpha-proteobacteria. [13] Thus in the Viral Eukaryogenesis theory, the ancestor of the mitochondria was an alpha-proteobacteria that existed in a syntrophic relationship with the archaeal ancestor of the eukaryotic cytoplasm.

5. A viral ancestor of the eukaryotic nucleus

The viral ancestor of the nucleus is proposed to have been an ancient member of the NCLDV viruses that infected the archaeal ancestor of the eukaryotic cytoplasm. [30] In the initial presentation of the theory, [20] a pox-like virus was chosen as a symbiotic ancestor of the nucleus because they, like the eukaryotic nucleus, possess large double stranded DNA genomes. [20] In addition to the large ds DNA genome, the poxviruses, possess several other features that are common to the eukaryotic nucleus. [20] They possess tandem DNA repeats at their telomeres, they encode DNA polymerases that are homologous to eukaryotic polymerases, they replicate in their host cell cytoplasm, they are membrane bound, and critically, they encode their own apparatus required to cap and polyadenylate mRNA prior to extrusion into the host cytoplasm, [20] a process that is otherwise only known to be performed by the eukaryotic nucleus and a range of other viruses.

In the years since the original Viral Eukaryogenesis hypothesis was published, it was found that the pox-like viruses are actually members of a larger grouping of viruses, the NCLDV viruses. [31] Included amongst the NCLDV group of viruses are the relatively newly described giant viruses, the Mimivirus, Mamavirus, Megavirus and CroV viruses. These large viruses have genomes larger than the smallest bacterial genomes. [22] Furthermore, phylogenomic analysis of the NCLDV viruses appears to show that they are ancient, emerging from the archaeal branch shortly before the eukaryotes originated. [17, 18, 19] Phylogenetic analysis of several specific genes, including the mRNA capping enzymes and DNA polymerases, place the genes of the NCLDV viruses at the base of the eukaryotic radiation, suggesting that they differentiated shortly before the eukaryotes evolved, and that they contain genes that are phylogenetically related to those that are used by the eukaryotic nucleus, [20, 32] Since mRNA capping is not observed in either bacteria or archaea, but is observed in NCLDV viruses it is argued that mRNA capping is a viral invention which ensured preferential translation of viral mRNA, and this feature has been passed on to its nuclear descendent. Significantly, NCLDV viruses such as the Mimivirus also possess their own highly divergent cap binding protein EIF4E which appears to be endogenous to the virus, and not obtained from the *Acanthamoeba* host. [33, 34] It therefore appears that the Mimivirus, like the eukaryotic nucleus, has its own DNA directed RNA polymerase, its own mRNA capping enzyme, and its own cap binding protein (eIF4E) to ensure translation of the viral transcripts by the host ribosomes. If the Viral Eukaryogenesis theory is valid these three sets of genes were present in the ancient NCLDV ancestor and allowed the virus to take over the translational apparatus in the host archaeon by directing the host ribosomes to recognise the viral mRNA which was differentiated from the typical uncapped prokaryotic host mRNA. In the process of taking over the transcription/translational regime, the virus re-organised the prokaryotic transcription/translation regime into the typical eukaryotic one where mRNA is capped prior to extrusion into the cytoplasm where the cap binding protein directs translation of the capped mRNA.

In addition to the discovery of the Mimivirus and related giant viruses, recent research into the *Acanthamoeba*, the host of the Mimivirus, illustrates the kind of 'community of organisms' proposed in the Viral Eukaryogenesis theory. In this case, it has been shown that *Acanthamoeba* is not just the host for the Mimivirus, it is also the host of many bacteria and viruses and where it acts as a kind of melting pot for the horizontal transfer of genes between bacteria and viruses. [35] Thus the *Acanthamoeba* cytoplasm can be the host of a variety of bacteria, as well as a variety of complex NCLDV viruses including the Mimivirus and Marseillesvirus, and that these 'invaders' can and do exchange genes with each other. It is proposed in the Viral Eukaryogenesis theory that the *Acanthamoeba* is a modern organism that represents a direct descendent of the kind of community that evolved into the eukaryotic cell. In terms of the Viral Eukaryogenesis theory, this community can be considered to be an 'ecosystem' of sorts containing a variety of independently derived 'organisms', some of which, like the mitochondria and nucleus are permanently linked to the single host, whereas others like the bacteria and Mimivirus are transient members of the ecosystem and capable of being transferred between communities by infecting new hosts.

5.1. The origin of meiosis and the eukaryotic cell cycle according to the Viral Eukaryogenesis theory

According to the Viral Eukaryogenesis theory, the three lineages that make up the modern eukaryotic cell originally replicated independently of each other, and due to natural selection, they eventually evolved to have the co-ordinated replication cycles seen today. [24, 36] In the process of evolution, it is proposed that the mechanisms of viral and cellular replication were exapted into the eukaryotic cell cycle.

In the case of the mitochondria, it is relatively simple to envisage a situation whereby the alpha-proteobacterial endosymbiont evolved its replication cycle to ensure that there were always several endosymbionts per cell, and thus it was highly likely that any daughter cells would posses at least one copy of the mitochondria. In the case of the viral lysogen there were more options available since viruses have evolved several complex mechanisms by which they are either maintained within a host (lysogeny) or transfer themselves to new hosts (infection). It is proposed that the mitotic cycle of the eukaryotes evolved from the mechanisms by which the virus established a permanent lysogenic presence in the host cell, [24] and that the meiotic cycle and sex arose from the mechanisms by which the virus transferred itself to new hosts.

5.2. Mitosis

Observations of modern viruses demonstrate that viruses can be maintained indefinitely within a host lineage either by integrating into the host genome like lambda or replicating as a stable low copy plasmid like lysogen in the host cytoplasm like P1. [37] Where a virus integrates into the host chromosome, its replication and stability are ensured by the host genome's mechanisms of replication and transfer to daughter cells. However, where a virus replicates as a plasmid-like lysogen, the virus must provide mechanisms to ensure its own replication and stable transfer to all daughter cells. In the case of the P1 phage, it has been found that the virus has a complex mechanism to ensure that the viral genome is replicated and maintained at a low copy number. [38] It is thought that keeping a low copy number is crucial to ensure that the metabolic burden of maintaining the virus is limited, so that the host is not at a competitive disadvantage when compared with hosts that have not been infected. [39] In addition to the mechanism to ensure a low copy number, the P1 phage has evolved at least two mechanisms to ensure that it is stably propagated to the daughter cells. [38] Firstly, the virus has evolved efficient partitioning mechanisms to ensure that a copy of the virus is mechanically segregated to each daughter cell before the daughter cells are divided. Secondly, the P1 phage has evolved a toxin/antitoxin mechanism to ensure that if the segregation fails to ensure both cells receive a copy of the virus, the cell not receiving the virus will die. This is achieved by having a long-lived toxin and a short-lived antitoxin that is continually produced by the viral genome [38] and is suggestive of the kind of mechanisms that viruses evolve to ensure that the viral lysogen is maintained indefinitely.

Studies at the molecular level on a variety of lysogens, such as other viruses (eg N15) and large conjugative plasmids such as F and R1 has shown that these low copy number lysogens have independently evolved similar, but non homologous mechanisms to ensure low copy number/ partitioning occurs as required. [40] In the systems studied at a molecular level, it has been found that copy number control is achieved by the possession of centromeric regions that perform several crucial roles. After the genome has been replicated there are two copies of the chromosome, both of which are 'handcuffed' together at the centromere region, which has the function of preventing further rounds of replication. [40] Subsequently when the cell is dividing, the centromere performs a second function, whereby it binds the proteins that are required to segregate the copies of the daughter chromosomes to daughter cells. [40] Once the segregation proteins are bound to the centromeres, the chromosomes are segregated via filament polymerisation to either pole of the cell. In the case of the R1 plasmid, these segregation proteins are closely related to the actin genes, [40] in other cases such as some of the large linear *Bacillus* plasmids they are be related to tubulin [41] and in the case of N15 phage and the F plasmid other classes of proteins are used. By segregating the chromosomes to either pole of the cell, the division of the host cell at the equator ensures both daughters obtain a copy of the chromosome, and the centromere is freed from the 'handcuffing' proteins, and thus free to enter into another round of replication. By this mechanism the copy number is kept low, and the viral chromosome is segregated efficiently to the daughter cells.

Several of the 'themes' of the replication of the large lysogens such as P1, R1, F and N15 are mirrored by the mechanisms controlling the replication of the eukaryotic chromosomes during mitosis and are thus consistent with the Viral Eukaryogenesis theory. [25] For example, the term centromere, representing a region of the chromosome that binds the two copies of the genome together, and representing the region to which the segregation proteins will bind and segregate the chromosomes to either pole of the cell is equally applicable to eukaryotic mitosis as it is to the segregation of lysogenic viruses and plasmids. The mechanism by which the chromosomes are segregated to either pole of the cell, i.e. via filament polymerisation, is also equally applicable to mitosis as it is to plasmid segregation and, amongst the range of proteins used by the lysogenic viruses and plasmids, there are tubulin-like proteins that are related to the tubulin used by eukaryotic cells to segregate chromosomes to either pole. [41] The evolution of mitosis in the eukaryotes is thus consistent with the Viral Eukaryogenesis theory in which the eukaryotic nucleus descends from a complex DNA virus that established a permanent lysogenic presence in its host. It is thus argued that the mechanisms by which the eukaryotic nucleus and chromosomes replicate and are segregated to either pole of the cell is a direct result of the descent of the eukaryotic nucleus from a large DNA virus [23] and arose directly from the mechanisms by which the ancestor of the eukaryotic nucleus maintained itself as a single copy lysogen in the host of the archaeon.

5.3. Meiosis and sex

In the Viral Eukaryogenesis theory, it is proposed that three general viral characteristics were exapted by the community to allow the evolution of meiosis and the sexual cycle. These three features were viral immunity, viral incompatibility, and viral infection, which when combined with the existing 'mitotic' copy number control mechanisms resulted in the evolution of sex and meiosis.

One of the viral features proposed to have been exapted from viruses in the evolution of meiosis and the sexual cycle is viral immunity functions. In the case of viral immunity, it has been observed that viruses often possess a mechanism to prevent multiple infection of a host by the same virus. For example, infection of *E. coli* by T4 bacteriophage immediately prevents further infection by other T4 viruses. [42] Similarly, the N15 virus (which lysogenises its host as a linear cytoplasmic prophage) possesses immunity functions that prevent lysogenised cells from being further infected by the N15 virus. [43] Conjugative plasmids, which share many features with lysogenic viruses, have also evolved immunity mechanisms which prevent donor cells transferring the plasmid to lysogenised recipient cells and these immunity mechanisms are well understood. [44]

Another critical viral feature exapted in the evolution of the meiosis and the sexual cycle is the viral/lysogen feature of incompatibility. Incompatibility can occur when a host is infected by two lysogens that utilise common copy number control mechanisms. This can occur because immunity functions do not in general prevent infection of the host by a different lysogen, and thus a host can potentially be infected by two lysogens at the same time. When multiple infections of a host by different lysogens occur, it is found that the lysogens are either compatible with each other, in which case they can replicate indefinitely in the same host cell, or incompatible with each other, in which case they will be segregated into separate host cell lines. [45] It has been found that compatibility or incompatibility of lysogens is dependent upon their mechanisms for replication and segregation. If they use non-homologous mechanisms, they are compatible, whereas if they use homologous mechanisms, they are usually incompatible with each other and thus cannot be maintained in the same lineage. [45] It is thought that the interaction between copy number control mechanisms, and maintenance of related but not identical lysogens would lead to incompatibility if a host was infected by two related lysogens which shared a copy number control mechanism.

Another critical feature exapted from viruses in the evolution of meiosis and the sexual cycle is proposed to have been the mechanisms by which the virus could horizontally infect new hosts. A critical feature of viruses (and plasmid lysogens) is that they can be transferred horizontally between hosts. In the case of viruses, the completion of the lytic cycle produces multiple virions that escape the cell and have many features that allow them to attach to and infect new hosts. In the case of lysogenic viruses, these viruses will enter the new host, and either establish a lysogenic cycle or enter a lytic cycle to produce more infectious virions. In contrast to viruses, conjugative plasmids do not have an extracellular stage to allow transfer from host to host within a population. Instead, these plasmids have evolved conjugation mechanisms that allow them to be transferred from an infected cell into an uninfected host cell. [44] In the case of the F plasmid, conjugation involves over 40 genes, including genes for pilus formation, surface exclusion, mating pair stabilisation, regulation and DNA mobilisation, [44] indicating that these processes are highly evolved and strongly selected for.

It is proposed in the Viral Eukaryogenesis theory that sex (syngamy) is exapted from the mechanisms by which the virus spread to new hosts. In this case, the virus either was produced as a free virion that used membrane fusion to enter new hosts, or the virus caused the host to conjugate with hosts that did not contain the virus. As shown in Figure 2 the virus/host would normally replicate via the lysogenic 'mitosis' like cycle in the hosts. However, under specific conditions, the host would produce new infectious viruses that could infect a new potential host that had not yet been infected by the virus. Once the new host was infected, the virus would enter into either the lysogenic (mitotic) cycle or enter into the lytic cycle to produce more infectious virions.

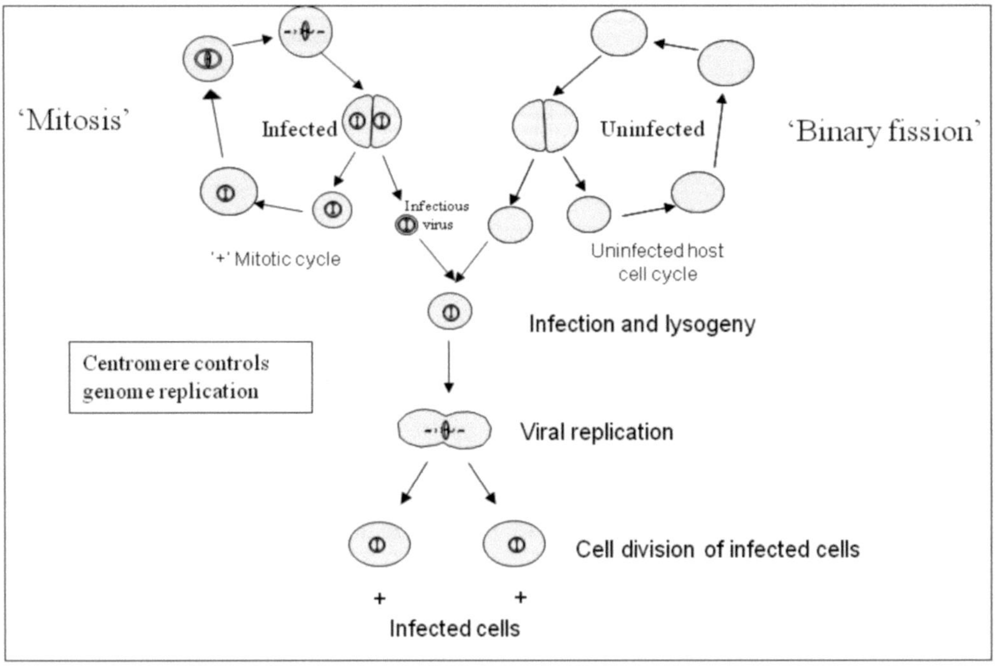

Figure 2. The lysogenic and infectious cycle of the viral ancestor of the nucleus. As shown, the archaeal ancestor of the eukaryotic cytoplasm initially replicated via a typical archaeal/prokaryotic binary fission style of replication (top right). However, when infected with the proposed viral ancestor of the nucleus, the virus maintained itself in the host using a mitosis-like process in which the copy number control of the virus was regulated through the use of 'centromere' sequences as is commonly observed in modern viruses and plasmids (top left). The virus could also enter into an 'infectious' cycle whereby an infectious virion would be produced that could infect new hosts that had not already been infected by the lysogen.

It is proposed in the Viral Eukaryogenesis theory that the eukaryotic sexual cycle evolved when two closely related but incompatible viral lysogens (designated 'a' and 'alpha') evolved from the original viral ancestor of the nucleus (Figure 3). When a cell infected by lineage 'a' encountered a host infected by lineage 'alpha', neither cell would recognise the other as being infected. As a result a virus could be transferred to a new host that already possessed a closely related lysogenic virus. Critically the two homologous but slightly different viruses would utilise the same mechanisms for copy number control. Once infected by the second related virus, the host would contain two viruses, and these viruses would be incompatible since they shared a common mechanism for copy number control. When the lysogens replicated, four viral chromosomes would be produced, and since they possessed homologous centromeric regions, the four chromosomes would be bound together by the 'handcuffing' proteins at their homologous centromeres. Once the four viral chromosomes were handcuffed together, the cells would be committed to go through two divisions before the centromeres were no longer handcuffed together. Only once the chromosomes were no longer 'handcuffed' together would the origins of replication be exposed, and the chromosomes be capable of entering into another round of replication.

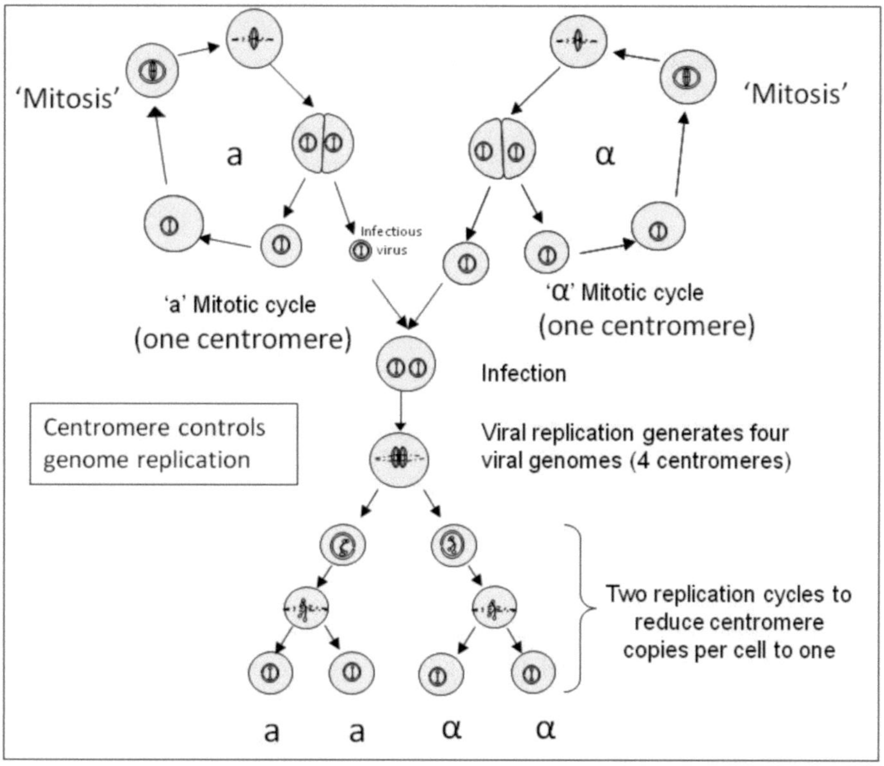

Figure 3. The eukaryotic sexual cycle arose when the lysogenic ancestor of the nucleus diverged into two closely homologous but not identical viruses utilising the same copy number control mechanisms. As shown two related viruses, designated 'a' and 'alpha' evolved that could maintain themselves in the archaeal host via the mitosis like lysogenic replication cycle. In this mitosis like cycle the copy number of the virus was maintained at unity by the use of centromeric regions. Since the two viruses were closely related to each other, they shared homologous centromeric regions, however the viruses were sufficiently different such that neither virus recognised the other virus as 'self' and thus a single host could be infected by both viruses. When an 'a' virion encountered a host infected by the 'alpha' virus, the 'a' virus would infect the 'alpha' host since it failed to recognise that it was infected already. As a result, both viruses would replicate, generating four homologous viral chromosomes that shared the same copy number control mechanisms. The four viral chromosomes would be then be 'handcuffed' together preventing further replication. The viral segregation mechanisms would ensure that the viral pairs would be segregated to either pole of the cell during replication. After a single round of replication there would still be two viral chromosomes attached to each other per cell and thus no further viral replication could proceed. As a result, the cell would have to enter a second replication cycle before the individual viral chromosomes could be segregated as a single copy into the host cells.

It is therefore proposed that the origin of sex and meiosis occurred when a complex DNA virus entered a new host via membrane fusion processes to produce a host containing two highly homologous, but not identical lysogenic viruses (Figure 3). Due to the incompatibility of the viruses, the next replication cycle of the cell would be a meiosis like cycle, using the same molecular machinery as the mitosis-like cycle. Thus the cell infected with the two homologous viral chromosomes would have to enter into a replication cycle in which the two viral chromosomes replicated once to produce four chromosomes, but the host cell would have to replicate twice, producing four daughter cells before the copy number control mechanism of the virus would allow the viruses to replicate again (Figure 3). The proposed cycle, based on the 'infectious strategy' of the lysogenic virus mirrors the eukaryotic sexual cycle, provides a mechanistic explanation for the reductive divisions observed in meiosis, and provides an explanation for why mitosis and meiosis share common themes and molecular machinery, yet result in quite different outcomes in evolutionary terms. [24] It also suggests that since mitosis and meiosis evolved at the same time, meiosis did not evolve from mitosis, and that the ancestral eukaryotic state possessed both mitosis and the sexual cycle.

6. Discussion

"The purpose of a scientific theory is to unite apparently disparate observations into a coherent set of generalizations with predictive power..... Historical theories, which necessarily treat complex irreversible events, can never be directly tested. However they certainly can lead to predictions. Even if this theory should eventually be proved wrong it has the real advantage of generating a large number of unique experimentally verifiable hypotheses. (Lynn Margulis, 1975)."8

Like the endosymbiotic theory for the origin of the mitochondria and the chloroplasts, the Viral Eukaryogenesis theory is an historical theory which treats complex irreversible events that can never be directly tested. Like the endosymbiotic theory for the origin of the chloroplasts and the mitochondria, it will be its ability to coherently unite apparently disparate observations, and make predictions that can be tested experimentally that will determine whether it is ultimately accepted.

If the radical concept of a viral ancestor of the nucleus can be entertained, then as shown in this chapter, the theory does unite a wide variety of disparate observations into a coherent set of generalisations. It can coherently explain many of the differences in genetic design between the eukaryotes and the prokaryotic bacteria and the archaea. For example, the origin of the nuclear membrane, the change from circular chromosomes to linear chromosomes, the invention of telomeres, the invention of mRNA capping, the invention of cap directed translation, the separation of transcription from translation, the invention of nuclear pores, the invention of karyopherins, are all a simple consequence of the evolution of the nucleus from a complex DNA virus that already possessed these features. That is, if it is accepted that a complex DNA virus like the Mimivirus evolved into the nucleus, there are no biologically

http://dx.doi.org/10.5772/56876

implausible steps required in the evolution of the eukaryotic nucleus since the Mimivirus is already membrane bound, possesses a linear chromosome with telomeres, caps its own mRNA, encodes its own cap binding protein (eIF4E), does not translate mRNA within its own virion, and exports its own capped mRNA into the host cytoplasm for translation. Thus the origin of the nucleus from a complex DNA virus has the potential to explain in a coherent fashion many of the dramatic changes in genetic architecture in the transition from prokaryotic to eukaryotic design. It also leads to testable predictions about the phylogenetic relationship between the eukaryotes, prokaryotes and NCLDV viruses. Although many of these testable predictions have not yet been tested, testing of some, such as the phylogenetics of the mRNA capping genes, have supported the theory. [20]

In addition to providing an explanation for the radical change in genetic design from the prokaryotes to the eukaryotes, the theory is one of the few theories for the origin of the eukaryotes comprehensive enough to provide a plausible explanation for the origin of the unique cell cycle of the eukaryotes. It predicts that the origin of mitosis, meiosis and the sexual cycle are all consequences of the very origin of the eukaryotic cell, and its viral derived nucleus. That is, because in the Viral Eukaryogenesis theory, the eukaryotic cell is actually a consortium of three phylogenetically independent members of a consortium, the eukaryotic cell cycle was by necessity quite different from any replication cycle of either cellular or viral organisms. Rather, the eukaryotic cell cycle that we see today is a synthesis of the replication cycles of three previously independent organisms, the nucleus, the cytoplasm and the mitochondria. Simply put, in the Viral Eukaryogenesis theory, mitosis is the mechanism by which the virus maintained itself as a single copy lysogen in the archaeal host, sex is the mechanism by which the virus transferred itself to a new host/ or the host was infected by new viruses, and meiosis is a natural consequence of the copy number control mechanisms being incompatible when two highly homologous viruses using the same copy number control mechanism infected the same host.

If the eukaryotes did evolve as proposed in the VE theory, a critical question to be asked is what made this new consortium uniquely capable of evolving beyond the comparatively simple 'prokaryotic world' of phages, bacteria and archaea and into the much more complex 'eukaryotic world' of complex multicellular organisms, and how did that evolution relate to the new modes of replication such as mitosis, sex and meiosis? It is the opinion of this author that both the new cellular design, where the 'cell' was uniquely compartmentalised into functionally specialised 'organelles' such as the mitochondria and nucleus, and the new modes of replication (sex and meiosis) were both critically important in the evolution of complexity in the eukaryotic lineages. In the case of the new cellular design it is proposed that the 'proto-eukaryotic' community eventually evolved into an amoeba-like eukaryotic ancestor that invented an unprecedented predatory life cycle that eventually lead to an evolutionary arms race in which the more complex and larger predators and prey had greater fitness. Critically however, the invention of sex and meiosis introduced a new mode of evolution, one that allowed the newly evolved eukaryotes to escape the limitations that Muller's ratchet imposes on prokaryotic evolution. In particular, the evolution of the 'meiosis' like cycle induced by infection with a second closely related viral lysogen allowed both repair of detrimental mutations within any one lysogen via recombination, and the spread of new advantageous mutations/genes that had evolved to increase the fitness of the viral genome, thus providing an immediate advantage to the consortium over its prokaryotic rivals. It is interesting to note here that when high mutation loads are deliberately introduced into viruses (including NCLDV virus such as poxviruses), the co-infection of a single host with multiple mutated virons allows the regeneration of functional viruses through a recombination process termed multiplicity reactivation (MR). [46, 47] This suggests that multiple infections of a single host by related viruses as proposed in the VE theory can side step the problem of accumulating mutational load seen with Muller's ratchet. As a result, the new meiosis like mode of replication allowed the integrity of the genetic information of the consortium to maintained at a higher level than seen in the prokaryotic world and this, combined with the new unique cellular organisation of the eukaryotes may have facilitated the evolution of complexity in the eukaryotic lineages.

The Viral Eukaryogenesis theory paints a radical new picture of the origin of the eukaryotes that would have been impossible to present even a few years ago. Prior to the 1970's symbiogenesis was scorned by the scientific community, despite the fact that today the evidence appears incontrovertible that the chloroplasts and mitochondria are symbiogenic in origin. Even the fact that there are three domains of life was only established with some difficulty by Woese in the 1970's, and the diversity of the Archaeal domain in particular has been expanded over the last 10 years or so to include phylogenetically new groups such as the Thaumarchaeota and Korarchaeota. The 21st century discovery of the hitherto unexpected giant viruses such as the Mimivirus have also shown that our knowledge of the natural biological world is still incomplete and most likely there will be more surprises in the future to challenge our accepted biological paradigms. Only time will tell whether ongoing scientific discoveries will prove or disprove the Viral Eukaryogenesis theory, but since we do not have an established paradigm that explains the origin of mitosis, sex, meiosis and the unique cellular architecture of the eukaryotes, it is perhaps time to entertain radical new theories for the origin of the eukaryotes, especially if they can be experimentally tested.

Author details

Philip Bell*

Address all correspondence to: philip.bell@microbiogen.com

Microbiogen Pty Ltd, N.S.W., Australia

References

[1] Malik, S.B., Pightling, A.W., Stefaniak, L.M., Schurko, A.M, & J.M. Logsdon, Jr. 2007. An expanded inventory of conserved meiotic genes provides evidence for sex in Trichomonas vaginalis. PLoS One. Aug 6;3(8):e2879

[2] Bell, G. 1982. The Masterpiece of Nature: The Evolution and Genetics of Sexuality

[3] Neumann, N., Lundin, D., & A.M. Poole. 2010. Comparative genomic evidence for a complete nuclear pore complex in the last eukaryotic common ancestor. PLoS One 8;5(10):e13241.

[4] Yutin, N., K. S. Makarova, S. L. Mekhedov, Y. I. Wolf, & E. V. Koonin. 2008. The Deep Archaeal Roots of Eukaryotes. Mol. Biol. Evol. 25(8): 1619–1630.

[5] Mereschkowsky, C. 1905. Uber Natur und Ursprung der Chromatophoren im Pflanzenreiche. Biol. Centralbl., 25: 593-604. (addendum in 25:689-691).

[6] Martin, W., & K.V. Kowallik. 1999. Annotated English translation of Mereschowsky's 1905 paper " Uber Natur und Ursprung der Chromatophoren im Pflanzenreiche". Eur. J. Phycol 34:287-295.

[7] noll, A. 2003. Life on a young planet: the first three billion years of evolution on earth pp 122-160

[8] Margulis, L. 1975. Symbiotic theory of the origin of eukaryotic organelles; criteria for proof. Symp. Soc. Exp. Biol. 29:21-38.

[9] Gray, M. W. 1999. Evolution of organellar genomes. Curr. Opin. Genet. Dev. 9(6): 678-87.

[10] DePriest, P.T. 2004. Early molecular investigations of lichen-forming symbionts: 1986-2001. Annu. Rev. Microbiol. 58: 273-301.

[11] McFadden, G.I. 1999. Endosymbiosis and evolution of the plant cell. Curr. Opin. Plant Biol. 2(6): 513-9.

[12] Keeling, P.J. 2010. The endosymbiotic origin, diversification and fate of plastids. Philos. Trans. R. Soc. Lond. B. Biol. Sci. 365(1541): 729–748.

[13] Emelyanov, V. V. 2003. Common evolutionary origin of mitochondrial and rickettsial respiratory chains. Arch. Biochem. Biophys. 420(1): 130-141.

[14] Bapteste, E., Brochier, C., & Y. Boucher. 2005. Higher-level classification of the Archaea: evolution of methanogenesis and methanogens. Archaea 1(5):353-63

[15] Csuros, M.,& I. Miklos. 2009. Streamlining and large ancestral genomes in Archaea inferred with a phylogenetic birth-and-death model. Mol. Biol. Evol. 26: 2087–2095.

[16] Pietilä, M. K., Laurinmäki, P., Russell, D. A., Ko, C. C., Jacobs-Sera, D., Hendrix, R.W., Bamford, D. H., & S. J. Butcher. 2013 Proc. Natl. Acad. Sci. U S A. Jun 3. [Epub ahead of print]

[17] Boyer, M., Madoui, M. A., Gimenez, G., La Scola, B., & D. Raoult. 2010. Phylogenetic and phyletic studies of informational genes in genomes highlight existence of a 4 domain of life including giant viruses. PLoS One. 2010 Dec 2;5(12):e15530.

[18] Nasir, A., Kim, K. M., & G. Caetano-Anolles. 2012. Giant viruses coexisted with the cellular ancestors and represent a distinct supergroup along with superkingdoms Archaea, Bacteria and Eukarya. BMC Evol. Biol. 12:156.

[19] Yutin, N., Wolf, Y. I., Raoult, D., & E. V. Koonin. 2009. Eukaryotic large nucleo-cytoplasmic DNA viruses: clusters of orthologous genes and reconstruction of viral genome evolution. Virol. J. 6:223.

[20] Bell, P. J. 2001. Viral eukaryogenesis: was the ancestor of the nucleus a complex DNA virus? J. Mol. Evol. 53(3): 251-256.

[21] Lang, B. F., Burger, G., O'Kelly, C. J., Cedergren, R., Golding, G. B., Lemieux, C., Sankoff, D., Turmel, M., & M. W, Gray. 1997. An ancestral mitochondrial DNA resembling a eubacterial genome in miniature. Nature. 387(6632):493-497.

[22] Raoult, D., Audic, S., Robert, C., Abergel, C., Renesto, P., Ogata, H., La Scola, B., Suzan, M., & J. M. Claverie. 2004. The 1.2-megabase genome sequence of Mimivirus. Science. 306(5700):1344-50.

[23] Ogata, H., La Scola, B., Audic, S., Renesto, P., Blanc, G., Robert, C., Fournier, P. E., Claverie, J. M., & D. Raoult. Genome sequence of Rickettsia bellii illuminates the role of amoebae in gene exchanges between intracellular pathogens. PLoS Genet. 2006 May;2(5):e76

[24] Bell, P. J. 2006. Sex and the eukaryotic cell cycle is consistent with a viral ancestry for the eukaryotic nucleus. J. Theor. Biol. 243(1): 54-63.

[25] Searcy, D. G., Stein, D. B., & G. R. Green. 1978. Phylogenetic affinities between eukaryotic cells and a thermophilic mycoplasma. Biosystems. (1-2):19-28.

[26] Margulis, L. 1996. Archaeal-eubacterial mergers in the origin of Eukarya: phylogenetic classification of life. Proc. Natl. Acad. Sci. U S A. 93(3):1071-6.

[27] Rose, C. S. & S. J. Pirt. 1981. Conversion to fatty acids and methane: Role of two mycoplasmal agents. J. Bacteriol. 147: 248-252

[28] Caldwell, S. L., Laidler, J. R., Brewer, E. A., Eberly, J. O., Sandborgh, S. C., & F.S. Colwell. 2008 Anaerobic oxidation of methane: mechanisms, bioenergetics, and the ecology of associated microorganisms. Environ. Sci. Technol. 42(18):6791-6799.

[29] Lang, B. F., M. W. Gray & G. Burger. 1999. Mitochondrial genome evolution and the origin of eukaryotes. Annu. Rev. Genet. 33: 351-397.

[30] Bell, P. J. L. 2004. The Viral Eukaryogenesis Theory. *In* Origins Genesis, Evolution and Diversity of Life. J. Seckbach, Ed. 347-394. Kluwver Academic Publishers. Dortrecht.

[31] Iyer, L. M., Aravind, L., & E. V. Koonin. 2001. Common origin of four diverse families of large eukaryotic DNA viruses J. Virol. 75(23):11720-34.

[32] Villarreal, L. P. & V. R. DeFilippis. 2000. A hypothesis for DNA viruses as the origin of eukaryotic replication proteins. J. Virol. 74: 7079-7084.

[33] Saini, H. K., & D. Fischer. 2007. Structural and functional insights into Mimivirus ORFans BMC Genomics. 8: 115.

[34] Jagus, R., Bachvaroff, T. R., Joshi, B., & A. R. Place. 2012. Diversity of Eukaryotic Translational Initiation Factor eIF4E in Protists. Comp. Funct. Genomics. 2012:134839.

[35] Boyer M, et al., 2009. Giant Marseillevirus highlights the role of amoebae as a melting pot in emergence of chimeric microorganisms. Proc Natl Acad Sci U S A. 2009 Dec 22;106(51):21848-53.

[36] Bell, P. J. 2009. The viral eukaryogenesis hypothesis: a key role for viruses in the emergence of eukaryotes from a prokaryotic world environment. Ann. N. Y. Acad. Sci. 1178: 91-105.

[37] Casjens, S. R. et al. 2004. The pKO2 linear plasmid prophage of Klebsiella oxytoca. J. Bacteriol. 186: 1818-1832.

[38] Łobocka, M. B. et al. 2004. Genome of bacteriophage P1. J. Bacteriol. 186(21): 7032-7068.

[39] Chattoraj, D. K. 2000. Control of plasmid DNA replication by iterons: no longer paradoxical. Mol. Microbiol. 37(3):467-476.

[40] Ebersbach, G. & K. Gerdes. 2005. Plasmid segregation mechanisms. Annu. Rev. Genet. 39: 453- 479.

[41] Chen, Y. & H. P. Erickson. 2008. In vitro assembly studies of FtsZ/tubulin-like proteins (TubZ) from Bacillus plasmids: evidence for a capping mechanism. J. Biol. Chem. 283(13): 8102-8109.

[42] Lu, M. J., & U. Henning. 1989. The immunity (imm) gene of Escherichia coli bacteriophage T4. J. Virol. 63: 3472-3478.

[43] Ravin, N. V., 2003. Mechanisms of replication and telomere resolution of the linear plasmid prophage N15. FEMS Microbiol. Lett. 221: 1-6.

[44] Frost, L. S., Ippen-Ihler, K., & R. A. Skurray. 1994. Analysis of the sequence and gene products of the transfer region of the F sex factor. Microbiol. Rev. 58: 162-210.

[45] Novick, R. P., 1987. Plasmid incompatibility. Microbiol. Rev. 51: 381-395.

[46] Abel, P., 1962. Multiplicity reactivation and marker rescue with vaccinia virus. Virology. 17:511-9.

[47] Mattle, M. J., & T. Kohn. 2012. Inactivation and tailing during UV254 disinfection of viruses: contributions of viral aggregation, light shielding within viral aggregates, and recombination. Environ Sci Technol. 46(18):10022-30.

Section 3

Teaching Meiosis

Chapter 5

Teaching of Meiosis and Mitosis in Schools of Developing Countries: How to Improve Education with a Plant Reproduction Project

Erica Duarte-Silva, Adriano Silvério and
Angela M. H. D. Silva

Additional information is available at the end of the chapter

http://dx.doi.org/10.5772/56929

1. Introduction

Recent investigations on Biology Education in Brazil showed that most classes involve the use of textbooks and illustrations [1, 2]. Theoretical and lecture classes predominate in Sciences and Biology courses [3, 4], and there is a scarce variety of teaching materials. On the other hand, recent investigations have led to the development of several practical lessons to improve education quality. Some studies involve proposals of biological models [5]; elaboration of teaching games [6]; analysis of biological specimens [7]; laboratory lessons using microscopy [8]; ecotourism in natural ecosystems, observation of wildlife and environment [9] and visits to Natural History Museums, Zoo and Botanical Gardens [3]. Moreover, other initiatives to improve theoretical classes of Biology and Sciences include donation of small libraries to rural public schools [10] and availability of computer with internet access in rooms at schools [11].

The Brazilian Basic Education system is divided into three cycles, as follows: *Educação Infantil*; *Ensino Fundamental* and *Ensino Médio*. *Educação infantil* can be translated here into Early Child Education [21], encompassing children from 0 to 5 years old; *Ensino fundamental* corresponds to Junior High School [4], for students aged 6 to 14 years old; and *Ensino Médio* corresponds to High School of United States of America (USA). In Brazilian High School, the students are teenagers from 15 to 17 years old. Nowadays, technology courses in Brazil are offered concomitantly with High School. Students that have access to Graduation courses enter higher education institutions after High School. Until the present moment, of all governmental and non-governmental programs to improve Brazilian Basic Education, the only one that became universal is the free distribution of textbooks in public schools [12,13] followed by the availability of computer with internet access at schools. These are present in 93.4% of High Schools; 70% of Junior High Schools and 30% of Early Childhood Education Schools.

Therefore, the present study is aimed to elaborate a project with practical lessons of Mitosis and Meiosis, at very little to no costs, based on the local environment of students from two cities of the Southeastearn Region of Brazil: São Mateus, in the state of Espírito Santo and Santos Dumont, in the state of Minas Gerais.

We proposed practical lessons of Mitosis and Meiosis within the context of a project of Plant Reproduction. The project bears the following contents: biological species; varieties; cultivars; gene; mutation; chromosome; ploidy; plant cell; cell division; mitosis; plant tissues; meristems; plant growth; plant asexual reproduction; meiosis; pollen and spores; plant sexual reproduction; plant life cycle; environmental education, effects of climate changes on plant reproduction and food security. These contents are consistent with textbooks of Biology, as well as with the National Curriculum Parameters for Sciences, Biology and Environmental Education [14,15,16,17].

The Plant Reproduction project is based on the local environment of the students, e.g., the plant material is based on species used as local food and crops cultivated in rural areas of São Mateus and Santos Dumont. Some of these plants are not native [18] and their introduction in Brazil is also described. Also, the historic deforestation process occurred in Brazil following to develop the several existing crops was discussed. The cities São Mateus-ES and Santos Dumont-MG are situated in the Atlantic Tropical Forest Biome, one of the world biodiversity hotspots [19].

According to Paulo Freire: an education adapted to real-life contexts of students, their environment and culture facilitates the learning process. Education can prepare students to become responsible citizens that will be able to promote positive changes in their society and their natural space in the future [20].

2. Teaching of meiosis and mitosis in developing countries: How to improve education with a plant reproduction project

The current project concerns the elaboration of practical lessons of Mitosis and Meiosis based on the local environment of teachers and students from two cities of Southeastearn Brazil: São Mateus-ES and Santos Dumont-MG. The costs of the project range from little to no costs. Also, the project can be adopted in developing countries.

A brief Environmental Analysis of São Mateus-ES and Santos Dumont-MG was conducted [22]. A literature review of São Mateus and Santos Dumont was performed, which included historical aspects, geographical characterization and the anthropic use of space. The literature review bears historical aspects of São Mateus and Santos Dumont from the time Brazil was a colony of Portugal (16th century) to the present time. The geographical characterization comprised: location, geomorphology, climate, hydrography, natural ecosystems and flora. Field work was carried out in tourist places and rural areas of both cities and aspects of

http://dx.doi.org/10.5772/56929

anthropic use of natural areas were investigated. Moreover, visits to historic markets, supermarkets and restaurants were conducted last year, and information on the local typical food was obtained. Pictures were taken of the major crops grown by the local population. Field work was carried out on secondary roads of both cities to record the main crops grown. Pictures of different sites were taken.

Based on data collected during the environmental analysis, vegetables that could be easily found by teachers and students were elected as material for the Project of Plant Reproduction. From May 2012 to January 2013, pictures were taken of macroscopic events related to mitosis and meiosis. Practical lessons of the microscopic events of mitosis and meiosis are also proposed, based on literature review of protocols, at little cost.

Biology textbooks published in Brasil were analyzed [14] as well as the National Curriculum Parameters for Sciences, Biology and Environmental Education [15,16,17] to understand how Mitosis, Meiosis and Plant Reproduction are being taught in Brazilian Basic Education. The Plant Reproduction project aims to raise the following question to students: How is a Plant life cycle? After understanding the main process of a plant life cycle, should the teacher motivate students to answer the following question: What is the relationship between Plant life cycle, Meiosis and Mitosis?

The present study is aimed to formulate biological pratical lessons to students from early childhood ducation to high school. However, Meiosis and Mitosis lessons are usually taught in the second half of Junior High School (for students aged 11 to 14 years old) and during High School (15 to 17 years old). In early childhood education and in the first half of Junior High School, some concepts of Plant life cycle are developed. As for the contents of the present book, macroscopic observations of plant life cycle could be used in all levels. Practical lessons of microscopy should be introduced at Junior High School and High School.

2.1. The plant reproduction project in the city of São Mateus, Espirito Santo state, Brazil

In the city of São Mateus-ES, we proposed a fieldwork at Guriri Beach (Figure 1A), one of the most popular tourist attractions in the city. Last year, students of São Mateus public schools have often visited that place, and, thus, we suggested that we could perform the proposed fieldwork during these annual tours. Teachers should encourage their students to bring zoom cameras; mobile phones with built-in digital cameras; magnifying glasses and hand lenses. Hand lenses are sold at cheap prices in Brazilian shops. Notebooks and pencils are also needed for note taking.

Guriri is an island in São Mateus. The road from downtown to the beach of Guriri bears some crops of the Dwarf coconut palm. The state of Espírito Santo, and, in particular, the city of São Mateus, are great producers of coconut water that is exported to tourist locations in Bahia, Espirito Santo and Rio de Janeiro. The dwarf variety contains sweet coconut water. Plant height facilitates harvesting. The Portuguese introduced the giant coconut palm in Brazil in 1533. The dwarf coconut palm came from Java, Malaysia, Cameroon and Ivory Coast and was introduced in Brazil from 1925 to 1978 [23].

The dwarf Coconut palm belongs to the same species of the giant coconut palm, *Cocus nucifera* L. Dwarf Coconut is a cultivar of *Cocus nucifera* named *Cocus nucifera* L. var. nana (Figure 1A-C). It is a mutation of the giant coconut palm. It has a mutant gene that prevents stem growth. This variety bears several cultivars of dwarf coconut: yellow of Brazil of Gramame (AABrG); yellow of Malaysia (AAM); green of Brazil of Jiqui (AVeBrJ); red of Brazil of Gramame (AVBrG); red of Cameroon and red of Malaysia (AVM) [23]. The dwarf coconut palm is abundant in Guriri Beach (Figure 1A-B). Students could take pictures of dwarf coconuts and listen to the teacher's explanation. In the subsequent class, at school, they should be encouraged to research about the concept of biological species; varieties; agronomical cultivars; chromosome, gene, mutation and mutant on their textbooks and educational websites. Regarding the exploration of the DNA concept, we suggest a low cost protocol of DNA extraction proposed by [7].

Besides Biology and Genetics, teachers could ask their students to search about historical and geographical aspects of São Mateus: e.g.: what kind of socioeconomic relationship existed between Portugal and Brazil in 1533? Has Brazil been an exploitation colony of Portugal from 22th April 1500 until 7th September 1822. When was the city of São Mateus founded? Was São Mateus founded during the period of coconut introduction in Brazil, in 1544 [24]. What is the geographical location of Java, Malaysia, Cameroon and Ivory Coast? Teachers of History, Geography and Portuguese should be invited to this tour and use transdisciplinary lessons.

The flowering and fruiting of coconut palm occurs throughout the year at 'the Restinga' vegetation of Guriri Beach (Figure 1A-C). The dwarf coconut can be used as material for the study of meiosis, mitosis and plant life cycle. Immature flowers can be explored to explain meiosis (Figure 1C). After pollination, flowers develop into fruits (Figure 2A-C). Coconut fruit bears several different tissues that can be seen with the naked eye (Figure 2B-C). These tissues grow during fruit development as a result of several mitotic divisions. In the field, the teacher can explore concepts of cell division and mitosis, and collect material to explore meiosis in a practical lesson in classroom.

The dwarf coconut palm is a monocot angiosperm. It belongs to the Arecaceae family, formerly known as Palmae family. The Life cycle of the coconut palm is a practical example of Angiosperm life cycle (Figure 1A-C and 2A-C), which is included in the curriculum of the Junior High School and High School. For a review of the theory of plant life cycle see [25, 26, 27, 28, 29]. Particularly about Angiosperm life cycle, there is an animation in [30].

All land plants, and some algae, have life cycles in which a multicellular haploid gametophyte generation alternates with a multicellular diploid generation [31]. In vascular plants, the dominant generation is the sporophyte [31]. This is an evolutive trend of vascular plants that include Pteridophytes, Gymnosperms and Angiosperms. If the sporophyte is the dominant generation, which visible structures of coconut palm belong to the sporophytic generation? All vegetative organs as roots stem and leaves belong to the sporophytic generation (Figure 1B). Some reproductive structures also belong to sporophyte, such as the inflorescence axis, sepals, petals, stamen, pistil and teguments of the ovule (Figure 2A).

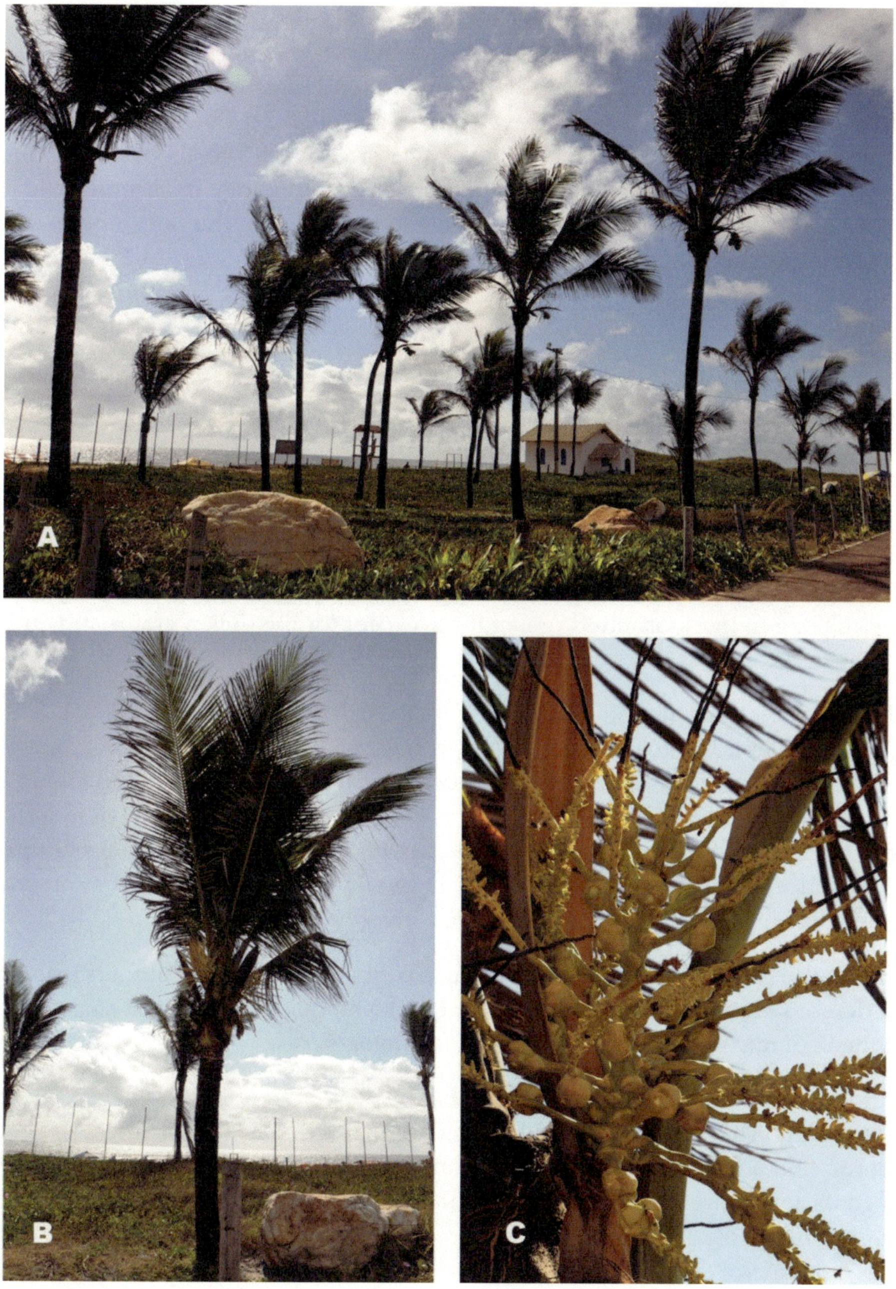

Figure 1. Guriri Beach at São Mateus-ES, Brazil (A) Guriri Beach. (B) The dwarf coconut palm. (C) Inflorescence of dwarf coconut palm with flowers and immature fruits.

The gametophytes comprise the pollen grains and the embryo sac. Pollen grains are produced within the anthers (Figure 2A). The embryo sac develops within the ovule. Pollen is the male gametophyte. The male gamete cells develop within the pollen grain. Male gametes are called sperm [24]. The embryo sac is the female gametophyte. The female gametes are: the egg cell and the middle of the cell. Almost all the following structures in the dwarf coconut can be viewed by the students: roots, stem, leaves, inflorescences, and flowers with sepals, petals, stamen and pistil (Figure 1B-C, Figure 2A). In classroom, with textbooks and educational websites, students should be able to recognize flower morphology in coconut palm flowers (Figure 2A). Teachers can cut anthers with a blade and observe the pollen grains. Students should observe pollen with hand lens or microscope. To prepare this lesson, the teacher collects some flowers and keeps them inside a sealed plastic pot with a spoonful of water under refrigeration at 4-8°C.

And how about learning how sporophytes give rise to gametophytes? In immature flowers or buds, the sporophyte gives rise to two types of sporangia: the microsporangium in the immature anthers and the megasporangium inside the immature ovule [24]. Microsporangium and megasporangium give rise to microspores and megaspores by meiosis. During meiosis, each diploid cell suffers a reduction division and gives rise to four haploid cells; haploid microspores will give rise to pollen grains by mitosis; also by mitotic divisions, the haploid megaspore gives rise to an embryo sac with seven cells [24]. In short, all coconut palm structures belong to the sporophytic generation, except for the pollen grains and embryo sac that are the gametophytes.

Regarding meiosis, it can also be asked: what are the differences between animal meiosis and meiosis of land plants? Meiosis in animals gives rise to gametes. In land plants it gives rise to spores within the immature flower; these spores germinate and develop into gametophytes; the pollen grain and embryo sac [24]. Animal gametes are generated by meiosis and land plant gametes are generated by mitosis. Meiosis occurs in land plants in immature anthers with liquids; after the end of meiosis, anther parietal tissues absorb liquids inside the anther. Several events take place in the cell, and meiocytes are converted into pollen grains [24].

Students can use a blade to cut small flower buds containing immature anthers from different sizes. Different size of anthers can correspond, in some cases, to different stages of another development, of microsporogenesis and microgametogenesis.

Then, students can view with a hand lens or a microscope the presence or absence of liquids inside the anthers. The presence of liquids indicates meiosis If the meiosis process is completed, students can find a dry anther with pollen grains. If school has got a microscopy laboratory with reagents, teachers can formulate a laboratory practice to see meiosis phases: Prophase I, Metaphase I, Anaphase I, Telophase I, Prophase II, Metaphase II, Anaphase II, Telophase II, as well as cytokinesis and the tetrad stage [8]. Cytokinesis occurs at the end of meiosis and gives rise to tetrads at eudicots. At monocots, cytokinesis occurs after meiosis I and after meiosis II. After meiosis I, the teacher can find dyads and after meiosis II, tetrads. For a review of the process of meiosis see [24].

Still in Guriri Beach, during the observation of coconut palm, some *Apis melifera L.* honeybees act as pollinators of coconut palm flowers (Figure 2A). It can be seen that honeybee transports an amount of pollen in the honeybee pollen basket. Honeybees are not native from Brazil and

http://dx.doi.org/10.5772/56929

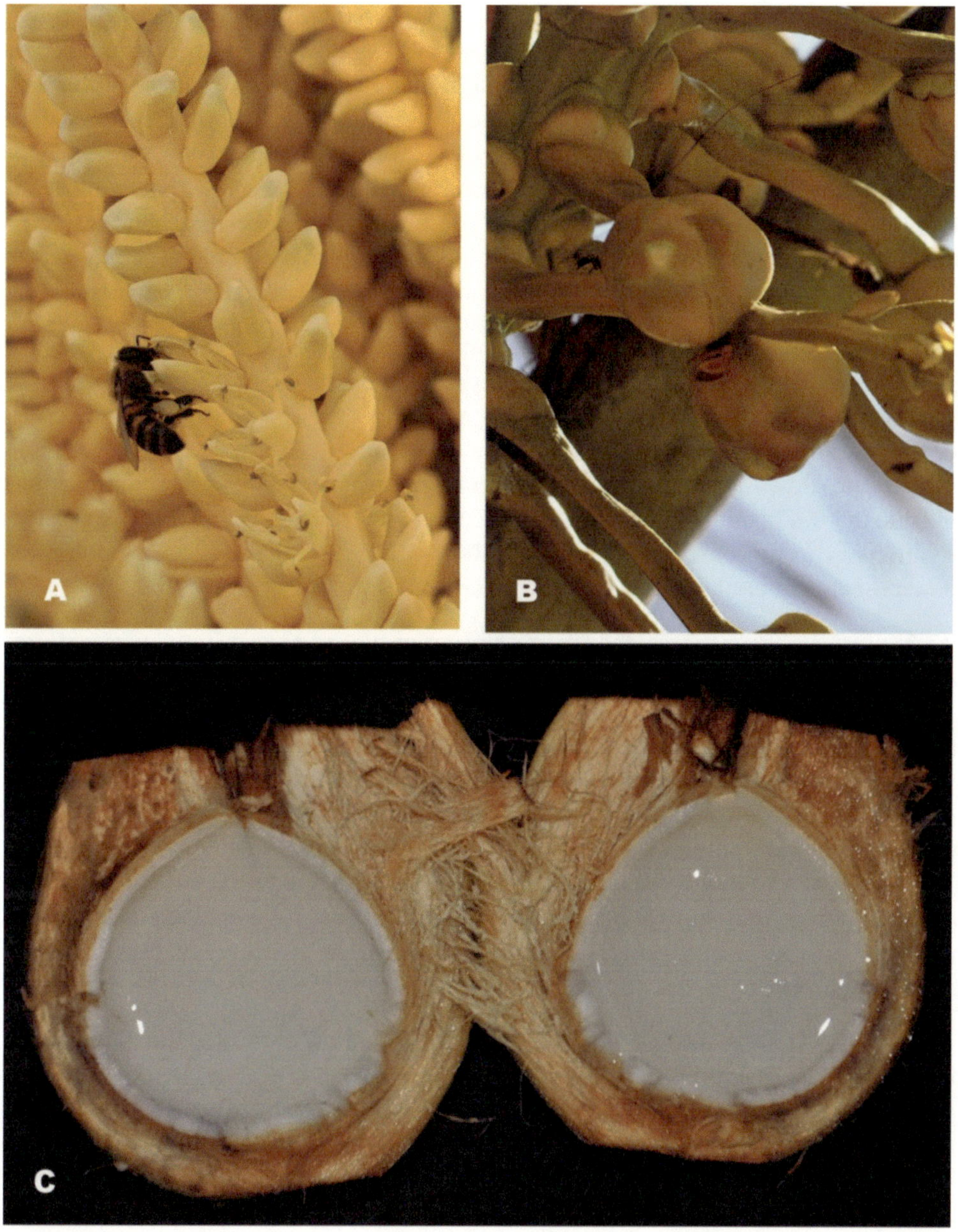

Figure 2. The dwarf coconut flower and fruit. (A) Immature buds of flowering and mature open flowers. See the pollinator on the open flower. (B) Immature coconut. (C) Mature coconut. Fruit pericarp, solid endosperm (edible part of the coconut) and liquid endosperm (coconut water).

are also known in the country as European bees. Honeybees were introduced in Brazil for honey production. Nowadays, the introduction of exotic pollinator species led to the extinction of native bees [32].

Pollinator agents transport pollen grains to stigma pistils and promote pollination. The pollination is the pollen tube growth along the pistil style carring the male gametes to the embryo sac, within the ovule. The fusion of male gametes with female gametes is called double fertilization. There are low-cost protocols for the observation of pollen tube *in vitro* growth that may be made at classroom with the presence of at least, one microscope [7, 33, 34]. Double-fertilization gives rise to embryo and endosperm (Figure 2C). The coconut water at immature fruit and the white coconut tissue at mature fruit stage compose the coconut endosperm. Figure 2C shows a fruit with coconut water and a little of solid endosperm. Animations about Double fertilization are avaible on [30]. A photomicrograph of double fertilization is disponible on [25].

At this point it is possible to formulate another question. How a small fruit containing this single seed with embryo and endosperm develops into a mature coconut (Figure 2B-C)? Embryo, endosperm, coconut seed integument as well as epicarpous, mesocarpous and endocarpous parts of the fruit suffer innumerable mitotic divisions to promote coconut growth. Protocol to observe chromosome of immature fruit somatic cells and mitotic divisions is available in [8]. Coconut water bears polythenic chromosomes [35] and can be used for the observation of chromosome morphology in schools that count on microscopy laboratory. To see how prepare material to analyse chromosomes see [8].

The native tree *Theobroma cacao,* the cocoa or cacao can also be used in the project involving meiosis and mitosis practical lessons. All the practical lessons on coconut palm which we suggested could be taught at Guriri Beach (Figure 1A-C, 2A-C) could also include cacao trees, abundant in farms of São Mateus-ES (Figure 3A-E). Chocolate is made from different proportions of cocoa nuts and milk. *Theobroma cacao* is an American native tree. In Brazil, *Theobroma cacao* occurs in Amazonia region, to the north of the states of Espírito Santo and Bahia. In farms, cacao is grown in some parts of the Atlantic Forest. *Theobroma cacao* also occurs in other tropical forests in Central and South Americas. During the Maya civilization, a territory nowadays situated at the Honduras and Mexico countries, *Theobroma cacao* was used to make a ritualistic drink. Cocoa nuts were transported to Europe after Spanish colonization came to American continent. In Europe, milk was added to this drink and the chocolate was invented.

The morphology of cacao tree is quite different from that of the coconut palm. Both species are angiosperms bearing flowers and fruits. The *Cocus nucifera* (Arecaceae family) is a monocot and *Theobroma cacao* (Malvaceae family) is a eudicot [35]. The morpholology of roots, leaves and flowers can be explored on field or at classroom. To keep lived plant material with good appearance, keep them at 4°C, in refrigerator, inside a sealed plastic bag with a spoonful of water.

According to the curriculum of botanical courses in Brazilian High School, after the study of diversity of vascular plants: Pteridophytes, Gymnosperms and Angiosperms, didactic books explore angiosperm plant anatomy [14]. A plant anatomy tissue closely related to mitosis is the meristem tissue [8].

The subsequent lesson concerns the following question: How is the development of morning glories? Where can the highest mitotic activity be found? Morning glory or *Ipomea purpurea* is an angiosperm, eudicot, from the Convolvulaceae family [36]. It Is abundant in anthropized

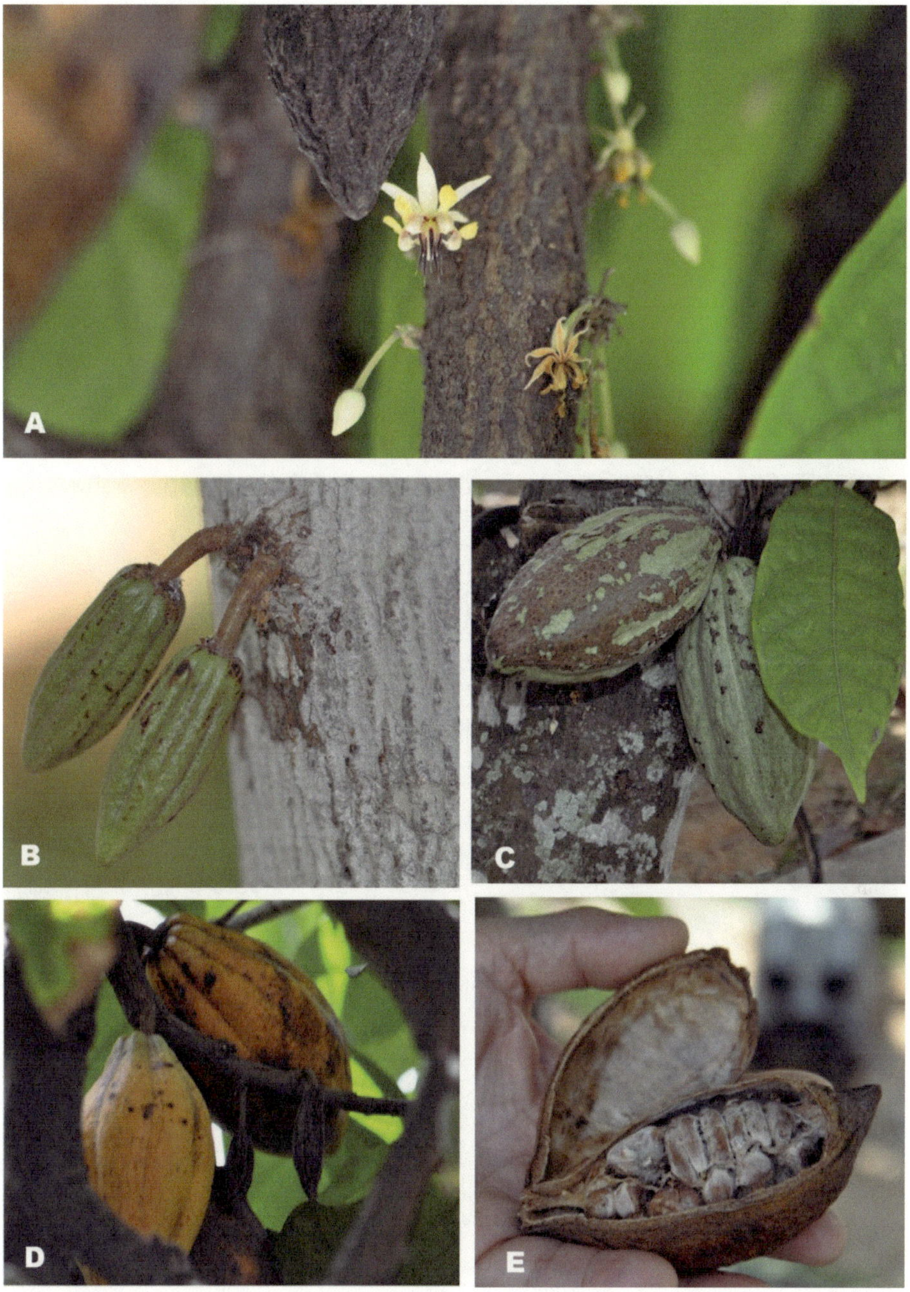

Figure 3. Cocoa tree. (A) Flower. (B) Small immature fruits. (C) Big immature fruit. (D) Mature fruit. (E) Seeds or cocoa nuts inside dry fruit.

environments of Restinga at Guriri Beach (Figure 4A). Morning glory occurs in the coastal regions of five continents and the colors of its petals range from white to purple [37]. Previous

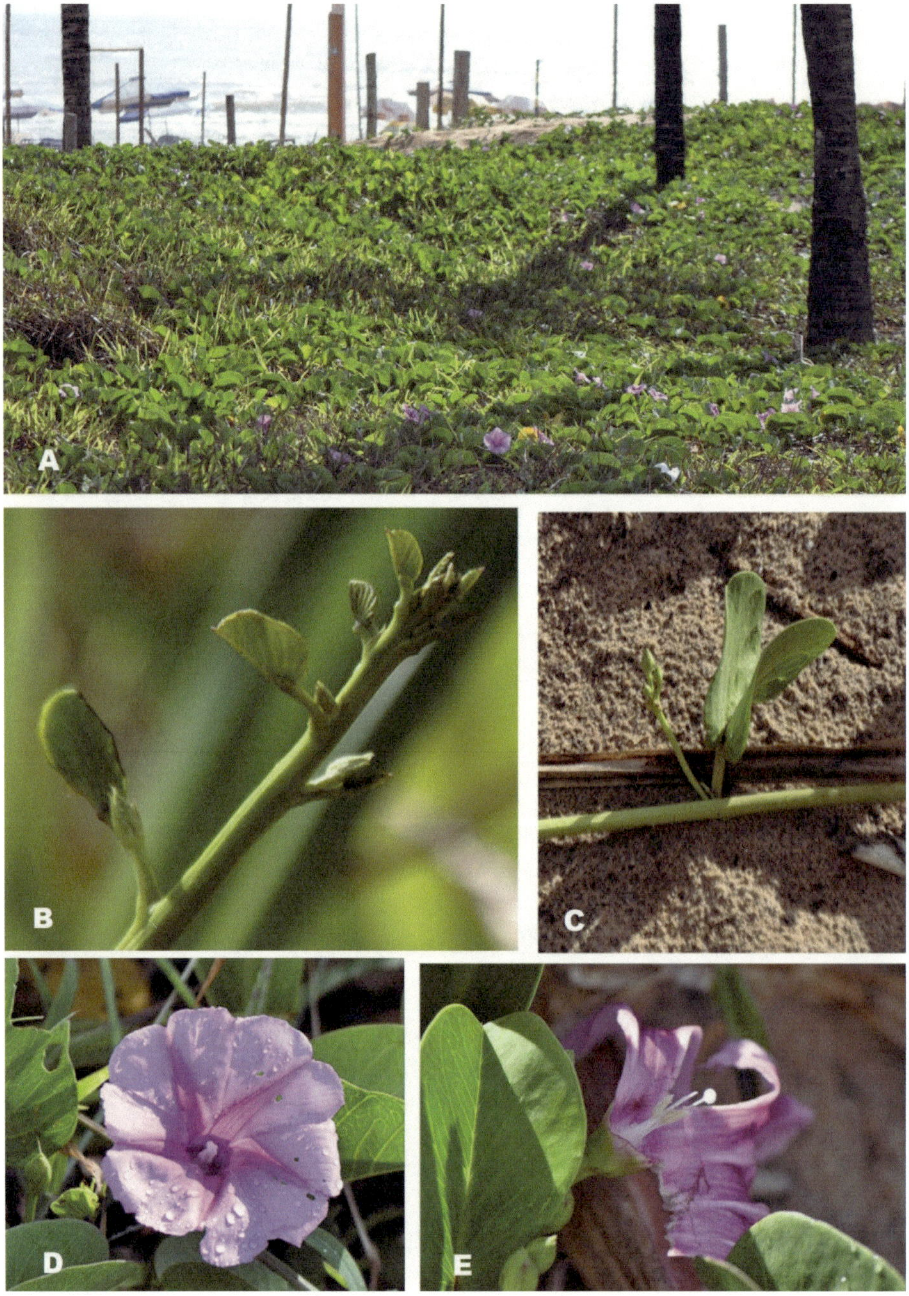

Figure 4. Morning glories. (A) Morning glory flowers at Guriri Beach, (B) Apical stem meristem. (C) Axilary flower meristem. (D) Open flower. (E) Stamen and pistil.

studies on morning glory polymorphism discussed the pollination natural selection that promotes genetic variability and, thus, different phenotypes with varied flower colours. Recent

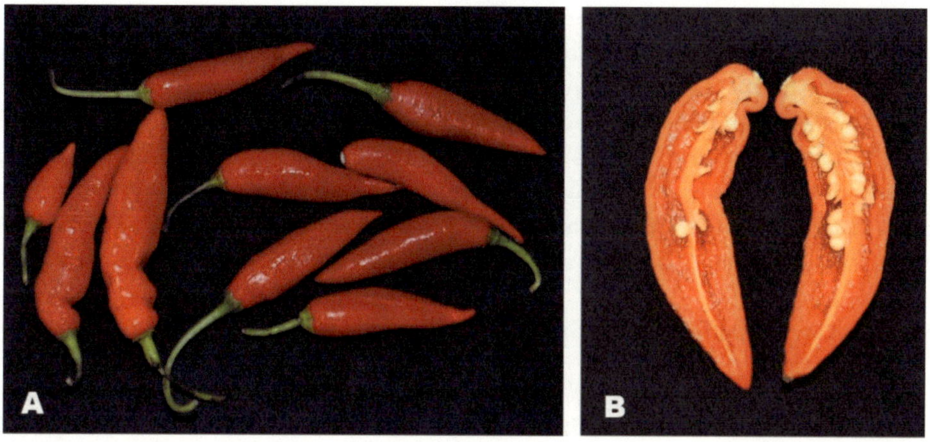

Figure 5. Brazilian peppers. (A) Pepper fruit. (B) Open pepper fruit showing seeds, the former ovule, or seminal rudiment.

studies revealed that the mutations underlying the genetic variation in flower colours were mostly caused by transposable elements. Restinga of Guriri Beach has morning glories with purple flowers and a small population with white flowers, nearby. This provides teachers with an excellent opportunity to explain pollination events and genetic concepts, their relationship with genetic variability, karyotype, genome, genotypes and phenotypes, and transposable elements. This lesson may be split into two parts: fieldwork at Guriri Beach and one lesson in classroom with the aid of textbooks and websites on the proposed concepts. Concernign Mitosis, let's go back to our questions: How is the development of morning glories? Where can the highest mitotic activity be found? Points of higher mitotic activity in plants are at meristems tissues. The growth of morning glories, as well as other herbaceous green plants, is a consequence of activity at the shoot apical meristem (Figure 4B) with elongation of shoots and axillary shoot meristem giving rise to leaves (Figure 4C) and flowers (Figure 4D). Flowers of morning glories can also be used for practical lessons on flower morphology, pollination and meiosis (Figure 4D-E) proposed above to *Cocus nucifera*, the coconut palm. Coconut palm and Morning Glory are interesting plant material for practical lessons in developing countries once these species have wide geographical distribution. Morning Glory is also a suggestion of plant material for explanation of Plant life cycle in Child Education. There is a DVD for small kids where morning glories are used in a germination experiment. In this experiment, children can view the lifecycle of the plant from germination to flowering [37]. Another suggestion concerns the observation of pollinator visitors in morning glories. This experience will involve the concepts of flower function, the pollination event and its consequences, the development of seed and fruits. To improve germination experiments, there is a detailed project of Sciences for Early Childhood Education at [38]. We also propose the study of plant life with germination experiments of bean, maize and pepper for all education levels Bean (*Phaseolus vulgaris*), maize (*Zea mays*) and peppers (*Capsicum* spp) are commonly found in Brazilian gastronomy (Figure 5A-B) [18]. The first event of germination is root or radicle emission. The apical zone of the root is situated in the root apical meristem. Following axial root development, axillary roots can develop by mitotic activity of the axillary region. Onions can be used in classroom to explore mitotic activity with root development. Big onions can be placed in a glass with water for a few days at room temperature. Long adventitious roots will develop inside the glass. Onion roots have large chromosomes and squash techniques can be used for their observation, as well as mitotic divisions [8]. In classroom, mitotic activity can also be demonstrated with bud growth at the stem of the potato (*Solanum tuberosum*), and leaf development in *Allium cepa*. Both biological materials show bud growth when kept in refrigerator.

2.2. The plant reproduction project in Santos Dumont city, state of Minas Gerais, Brazil

Santos Dumont (21°27′25″S 43°33′10″ O) is located in the state of Minas Gerais. The city was first called Palmyra until 1932 when it was named after the Brazilian aviation pioneer Alberto Santos Dumont [34], who was born in Palmyra, Brazil, in 1873 and died in 1932. The heir of a wealthy family of coffee producers, Santos Dumont dedicated himself to flying studies and experiments in Paris, France, where he spent most of his adult life [39]. Santos-Dumont designed, built and flew the first flying machine, demonstrating that controlled flight was possible [35]. This conquest of air, in particular the *Deutsch de la Meurthe* prize that he won on October 19th, 1901, in a flight around the Eiffel Tower, made him one of the most well-known figures of the world during in the early 20th Century [40]. In Brazil, he is considered the Father of Aviation and Patrone of Aeronautics. Moreover, there are several artistic monuments in his honour in Brazilian airports (Rio de Janeiro and Porto Alegre) and national parks (Iguaçu Falls). Three of the many houses where he spent his life are now historical places and museums, in Santos Dumont-MG (Brazil), Paris, Ile de France (France) and Petrópolis-RJ (Brazil).

To improve the teaching of Meiosis and Mitosis in Santos Dumont, we propose a fieldwork in the farm where Alberto Santos-Dumont was born, the Cabangu Historical Museum (Figure 6A-B) and its green area (Figure 6C). Santos Dumont is located in Serra da Mantiqueira, 850 meters above sea (Figure 6C). The climate is altitudinal tropical with dry and wet seasons [41]. The maximum annual temperature is 30°C and the minimum is 12°C [36] and heavy tropical rains are common at the end of the afternoons. The original vegetation belongs to Atlantic Forest Biome (Figure 6D) [19]. Most of the territory was deforested and replaced with coffee crops in the 19th Century. The old r crops of coffee no longer exist and the land is used for dairy cattle production (Figure 6E). *Araucaria angustifolia,* a Brazilian species of Gymnosperm is native of Santos Dumont. Despite of desforestation, *Araucaria* trees are kept in pasture (Figure 6F). They have economic importance. *Araucaria* seeds are used in local gastronomy.

The local climate favors the occurrence of Bryophytes and Pteridophytes (Figure 7A-B). Such specimens could be used to explain the diversity of land plants and the life cycle of land plants. Pteridaceae are native species (Figure 6D and Figure 7A) and can be found in local houses where they are used as ornamental plants (Figure 7B).

Finally, we select two common angiosperms of the region: the violet, one eudicot, and the banana, one monocot. Both plants cited are exotic; the first one is original from Africa, and the second one, from Asia.

http://dx.doi.org/10.5772/56929

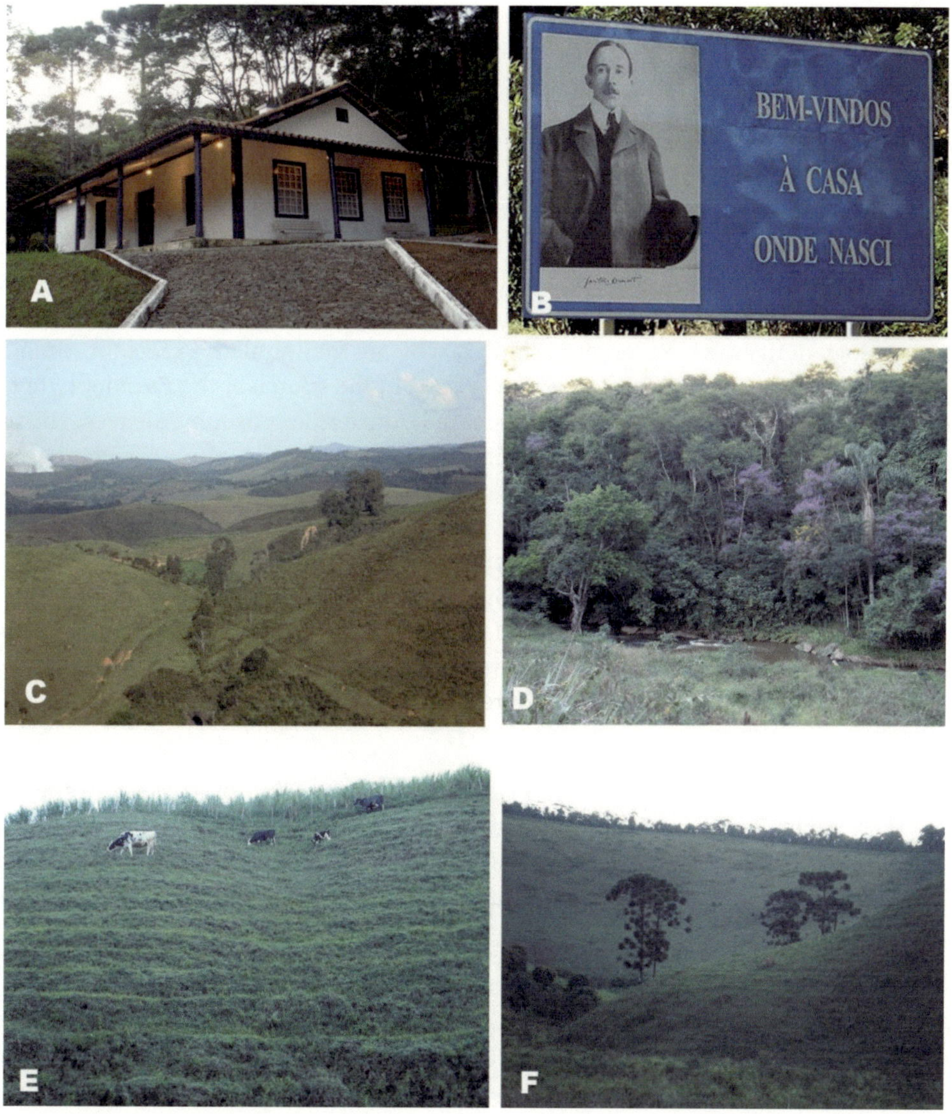

Figure 6. Landscapes of Santos Dumont city, Minas Gerais state, Brazil. (A) *Cabangu* Museum. House where Alberto Santos Dumont was born. (B) Alberto Santos Dumont photograph at Cabangu Museum. (C) Cabangu Museum. View of landscape from the top of mountain. (D) Original vegetation of Santos Dumont city. Atlantic Forest. (E) Cattle for dairy production. (E) The native gymnosperm *Araucaria angustifolia*.

We propose a fieldwork at Cabangu Museum with the purpose of observing the diversity of land plants. There are many *Araucaria* specimens near the House of Alberto Santos Dumont there. There is a waterfall behind the pavilion of Aviation where many species of Pteridophytes can be found. Walking from the Aviation pavilion until the playground area there are many Bryophytes at dry season. At playground area, there is the entrance of the heliport trail. At the beginning of this trail, we can find the *samambaia-açu* (Figure 7A), an arborescent Pteridophyte, an endangered species. It is a typical element of Atlantic Forest, used in past to produce plant pots named in Portuguese language as "xaxim". Nowadays, xaxim extraction is forbidden by Brazilian law code.

After the fieldwork, the teacher may propose a practical lesson of reduction division (meiosis) and plant life cycle in the classroom. The fertile leaves of pteridophytes (Figure 7B), pollen cones of *Araucaria* (Figure 7C), violet flowers and banana flowers (or any other angiosperm flower) must be collected and transported to the classroom. Using a hand lens or a microscope, observe Pteridophyte spores, *Araucaria* pollen, and angiosperm pollen. And then ask the students the following question: how is the morphology of the three materials? In conclusion, the morphology of the three materials is similar. Why are they similar? A meiotic diploid cell gives rise to four haploid spores, as it was observed in the spores of the Pteridophyte fertile leaves. During the Pteridophyte life cycle, spores fall from fertile sporophyte leaves. The spores germinate on soil, undergo many mitosis and give rise to a gametophyte which give rise to male and female gametes by mitotic divisions. Then, another question should be asked: Gymnosperm and Angiosperm pollen grains are spores? Reviewing part explained above, at page 4, Gymnosperm and Angiosperm pollen grains are male gametophytes that developed into sporodermis, the case of ancient spore. By mitotic divisions occurred inside sporodermis, the spore germinates and gives rise to a male gametophyte, in a endosporic mode. This fact explains why spores and pollen grains are so similar. Spores gives rise to pollen grains. At sum, Reduction meiosis gives rise to spores. Spores, by mitotic divisions, develop into gametophytes.

Gametophytes generate gametes by mitotic divisions. The fusion of gametes in the female gametophyte named embryo sac gives rise to seeds. There is an embryo within the seeds that will germinate and give rise to a new sporophytic plant and the endosperm, a kind of embryonic nutrition tissue. The fusion of gametes and the seed production is sexual plant reproduction.

Violets, bananas and grass species used for cattle forage are three local examples of reproduction for vegetative propagation (Figure 8A-G). Violets form other plants by budding in their leaves. Bananas and grass are monocots with underground stems. Their stems propagate giving rise to other plants. Mitotic divisions propagate these plants. They have the same ploidy of mother plant and the same genome. They are clones. It is a kind of natural cloning.

Genetic variability is promoted by crossing-over during meiosis that generates spores, and during the fusion of gametes, in sexual reproduction. Vegetative propagation does not promote genetic variability. It is a technique used in agriculture to homogenize crop population and, thus, has some advantages. On the other hand, clone populations are susceptible to diseases. They have the genome, and, consequently, the same immune system responses. The banana propagates spread out by vegetative propagation. Most banana populations do not have seeds, or else seeds are abortive. Many studies address the genetic variability of bananas and their risk of extinction. In classroom, teachers can place violets leaves inside glasses containing water to be observed by students: root budding will occur in violet leaves. At fieldwork, in students' houses and in the farms of Santos Dumont, teachers may ind out the banana shoots from the soil and grass to show how long can be a cloning population reproduced by vegetative propagation.

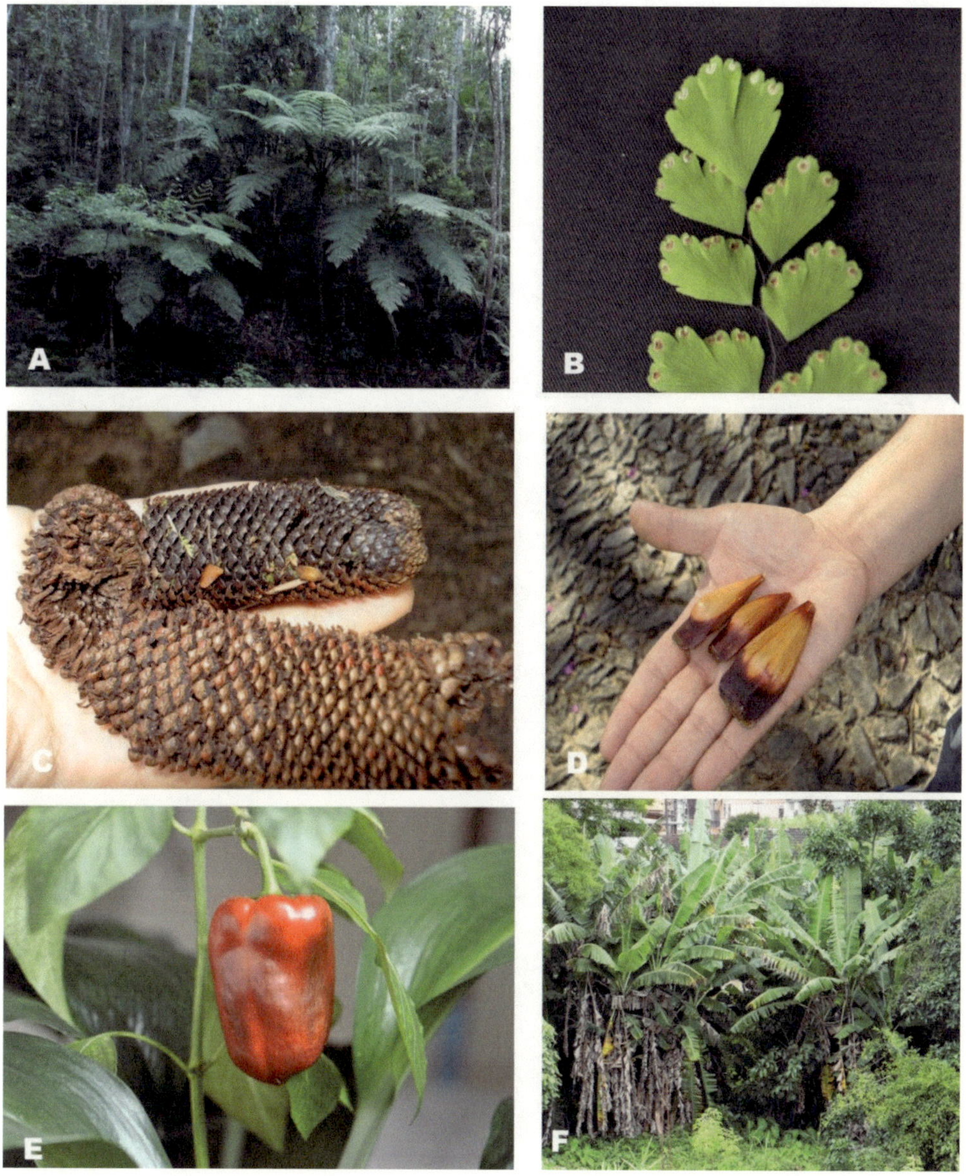

Figure 7. Diversity of vascular plants in the city of Santos Dumont, Brazil. (A) Pteridophyte. *Dicksonia* gender. called *samambaia-açu* in Brazil (B) Pteridophyte. *Adiantum* gender. called *avenca* in Brazil. (C) Gymnosperm. Pollen cones of *Araucaria angustifolia*, the *Pinheiro do Paraná*. (D) Seeds of *Araucaria angustifolia*, known as *pinhões*. (E) Angiosperm, eudicot. Pepper fruit. (F) Angiosperm monocot. Banana trees.

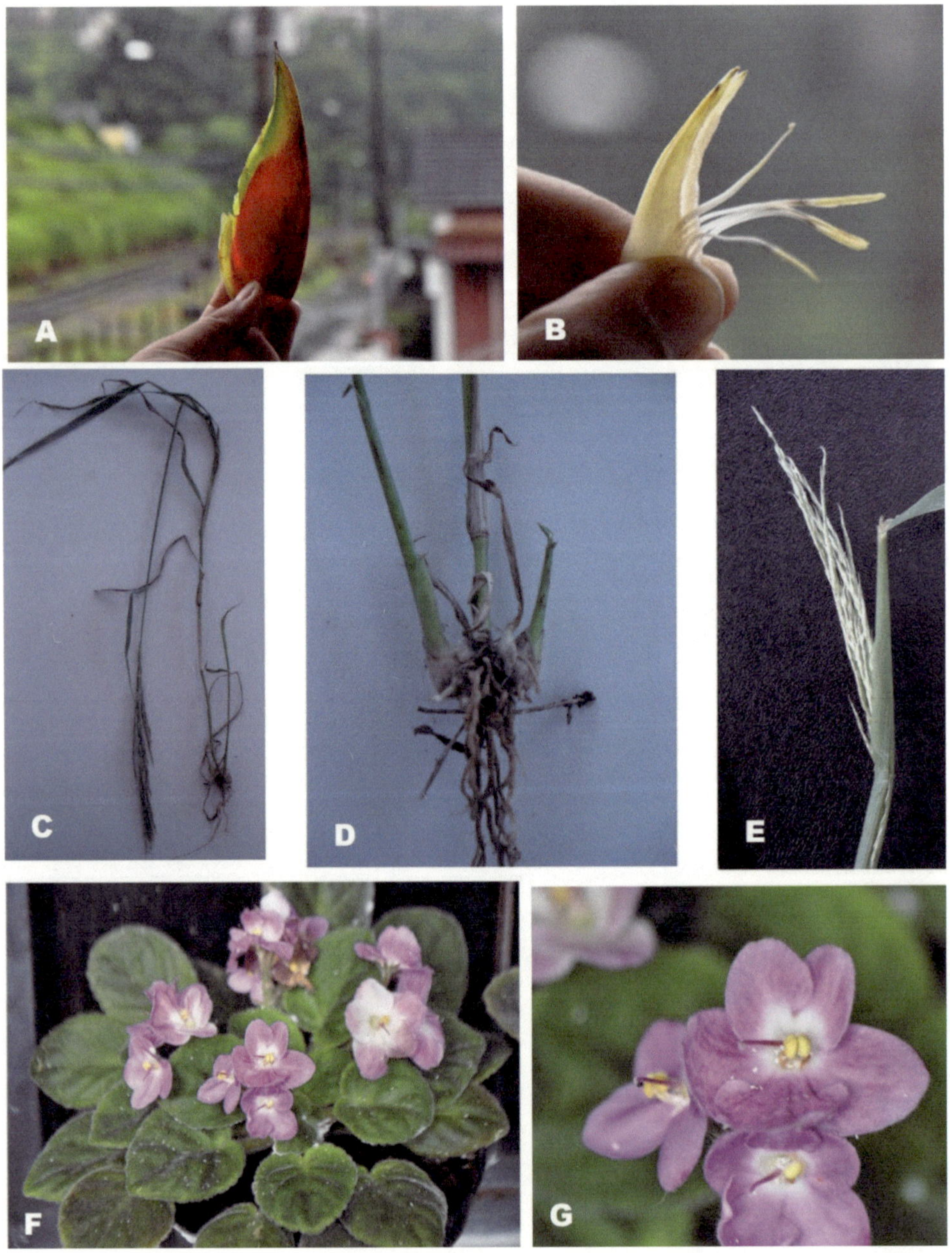

Figure 8. Eudicots and Monocots species that occur in the city of Santos Dumont, Brazil. Examples of vegetative propagation. (A) Monocot. Ornamental Banana. *Heliconia* gender. Red Bract. (B) Ornamental Banana. Flower. Stamen and pistil. (C) Monocot. Grass. Poaceae family. (D) Vegetative propagation on grass stem basis. (E) Inflorescence of grass. (F) Eudicot. Violet. Their leaves are able to do vegetative propagation. (G) Violet flower.

http://dx.doi.org/10.5772/56929

3. Conclusions

In the present didactic sequence of meiosis and mitosis lessons, we show different botanical materials from Brazil local environments. Dwarf coconut palm and cacao trees are two agricultural crops of São Mateus city, ES. Morning glories compound the Restinga of Guriri Beach visited by tourists throughout the year. Cocoa juice, bean, maize, peppers, potato and onion are part of the local gastronomy and are cultivated in small farms for sale and subsistence. The plants showed at the present work (coconut tree, morning glory, peppers, bananas and others) are present at beaches and crops of developing countries from Latin American, Africa, Asia and Oceania.

At the present chapter, there are many cited works at Portuguese and Spanish language, a benefic aspect to Developing Countries of Latin American, as well as the African nations of Angola, Mozambique, São Tomé and Príncipe, Equatorial Guinea, Guinea Bissau, Cape Verde islands; and the Asian areas of Macao and East Timor. On other hand, for teachers from other developing countries, we recommend the following educational references in English language [25, 52, 53, 54, 55, 56, 57, 58].

To produce coconut fruits, cocoa nts, beans and maize grains and peppers fruit plants reduction division (meiosis) is required. Meiosis generates spores that germinate and will develop into pollen grains and embryo sacs. Plants also need sexual reproduction through pollination, promoting the fusion of male and female gametes. The fusion of gametes or fecundation only occurs if the pollen tube grows through the style carrying male gametes inside.

Meiosis can be affected by temperature rise. Increase in temperature causes defective meiosis [41]. There are many consequences of defective meiosis, e.g. anomalous flowers with no pollen grains or pollen grains that fail to grow pollen tubes [41, 42]. The practical lesson of pollen tube growth [7], proposed here can show students if the plants studied bears viable pollen grains, as a result of a normal meiotic process. Based on this, plant reproduction is stressed by increase in temperature. Therefore, plants produce less seeds and fruits. Eighthy percent of the world edible plants depend on sexual reproduction for propagation [43]. That's why global warming may affect food production.

In the next 100 years, it is estimated that the global temperature will increase 1.4 to 5.8 °C [44, 45, 46]. Although the reasons behind global warming are still controversial, its adverse consequences are clear and are a matter of increasing concern worldwide [33]. Climate changes consequences include decrease in reproductive performance of plant species in natural biomes and crops [41, 44]. Studies of the effect of climate changes on plant breeding have been a trend in the international scientific scenarios of plant reproduction [45]. Studies on the effect of temperature on plant propagation were conducted with coffee, demonstrating that the global warming expected by the IPCC for our planet promotes the emergence of sterile flowers in coffee plants. The decrease in the number of flowers has reduced the number of coffee grains produced [44]. Some literature reviews cite temperature increases as one of the causes of pollen sterility [25, 41, 44, 45]. The sterile pollen grain is a structure that does not emit the pollen tube containing the male gametes, and therefore generates lower pollination and fertilization, causing a reduction in the production of fruits and seeds [25, 45]. The performance of pollen is an important factor for successful fertilization, but the high variability in pollen behavior in the same species occurs under many environmental conditions [47, 48], such as temperature, water stress, availability of nutrients, ultraviolet (UV) light quality and intensity, and CO2 concentration [47].

Likewise, seeds depend on the physiological conditions for germination, e.g. appropriate temperatures [41]. Above a certain temperature, both pollen grains and seeds are incapable of germination generating local extinctions of populations of native plants [33] or decrease in agricultural crops [42, 39].

Another type of plant reproduction is vegetative propagation, e.g., potato and cassava crops. The propagation of plants by cuttings generates clonal production [43]. Clones produced from a plant do not have the entire genetic variability from one species [49]. Sexual reproduction (natural or assisted) is needed for the preservation of the genetic variability of one species [50]. The phase of sexual reproduction in plants can be particularly vulnerable to climate changes [39].

The improvement of quality in meiosis and mitosis teaching is an opportunity to explore plant reproduction background that involves: Education for Food Security; Environmental Education and Education for Science and Biotechnology. In the last International Congress on Sexual Plant Reproduction, Food security was the central theme as the quotation below: food is required for survival; agricultural productivity expense increasing energy and water consumption; food shortages can soon be critical; a major drought; a natural disaster or war; greater climate instabilities now seem inevitable, and we know we cannot increase production by increasing energy input; global food security will demand the development and delivery of new technologies to increase food production on limited arable land, and without increasing the amount of water and fertilizers [41].

Acknowledgements

We would like to thanks Fundação Educacional São José by support the present research. We would also thank the anonymous referees for suggestions.

Author details

Erica Duarte-Silva[1,2], Adriano Silvério[1] and Angela M. H. D. Silva[1]

*Address all correspondence to: ericaduartesilva@gmail.com

1 Education College of Santos Dumont- MG (FESJ), Brazil

2 DCAB/ CEUNES/ Federal University of Espirito Santo, São Mateus, ES, Brazil

References

[1] Farias JG., Bessa E., Arnt AM. Comportamento animal no ensino de Biologia: possibilidades e alternativas a partir da análise de livros didáticos de Ensino Médio. Revista electrónica de las Ciências 2012; 11(2): 365-384. http://www.saum.uvigo.es/reec/lang/spanish/reecantiguo.htm (accessed 11 January 2013).

[2] Torres Santomé J. Livro texto e controle do currículo. In: Torres Santomé J. Globalização e interdisciplinariedade: o currículo integrado. Porto Alegre: Artes Médicas Sul Ltda. 1998.

[3] Vieira V., Bianconi ML., Dias M. Espaços não-formais de ensino e o currículo de ciências. Ciência e Cultura 2005; 57(4): 21-23. http://cienciaecultura.bvs.br/scielo.php?script=sci_issuetoc&pid=0009-672520050003&lng=en&nrm=iso (acessed 13 January 2013).

[4] Vasconcelos SD., Souto E. O Livro didático de Ciências no Ensino Fundamental – proposta de critérios para análise do conteúdo zoológico. Ciência & Educação 2003; 9 (1): 93-104. http://www.scielo.br/pdf/ciedu/v9n1/08.pdf (acessed 13 January 2013).

[5] Braga CMDS. O uso de modelos no ensino da divisão celular na perspectiva da aprendizagem significativa. MSc thesis. Brasília University, Brazil; 2010. http://repositorio.bce.unb.br/handle/10482/9069 (accessed 13 January 2013).

[6] Spiegel CN., Alves GG., Cardona TDS., Melim LMC., Luz MRM., Araújo-Jorge TC., Henrique-Pons A. Discovering the cell: an educational game about cell and molecular biology. Journal of Biological Education 2008; 43(1): 27-36. http://www.tandfonline.com/doi/abs/10.1080/00219266.2008.9656146 (accessed 13 January 2013).

[7] Santos DYAC., Ceccantini G. (org.) Proposta para o ensino de Botânica: curso de atualização de professores da rede pública de ensino. São Paulo: São Paulo University, Biosciences Institute, Botany Department. 2004. felix.ib.usp.br/posbotanica/index.php/extensao (accessed 04 March 2012)

[8] Guerra M., Souza MJ. Como observar cromossomos: um guia de técnicas em citogenética vegetal, animal e humana. Rio Preto: Funpec. 2002.

[9] Ramalho RRF. Inclusão do Turismo em programas escolares: uma proposta de preservação e valorização do meio ambiente e da cultura. Ateliê Geográfico 2009; 3(1): 60-82. http://www.revistas.ufg.br/index.php/atelie/article/viewArticle/6255 (accessed 13 January 2013).

[10] Empresa Brasileira de Pesquisa Agropecuária. Embrapa: Projeto Minibibliotecas. http://hotsites.sct.embrapa.br/minibibliotecas (accessed in 13 January 2013).

[11] Todos pela Educação: Artigo de 30 de julho de 2012. Menos da metade das escolas públicas de ensino fundamental têm acesso à Internet. http://www.todospelaeduca-

cao.org.br/comunicacao-e-midia/noticias/23529/menos-da-metade-das-escolas-publicas-de-ensino-fundamental-tem-acesso-a-internet/ (accessed in 13 January 2013).

[12] Martins L., Santos GS., El-Hani CN. Abordagens de saúde em um livro didático de Biologia largamente utilizado no Ensino médio brasileiro. Investigações em Ensino de Ciências 2012; 17(11): 249-283. www.if.ufrgs.br/ienci/artigos/Artigo_ID292/v17_n1_a2012.pdf (accessed in 30 July 2012).

[13] Rosa MA, Mohr A. Os fungos na escola: análise dos conteúdos de micologia em livros didáticos no ensino Fundamental de Florianópolis. Experiências em Ensino de Ciências 2010; 5(3): 95-102. if.ufmt.br/eenci/artigos/Artigo_ID124/v5_n3_a2010.pdf (accessed in 30 July 2012).

[14] Silva-Junior CD., Sasson S. Biologia: volume único. São Paulo: Saraiva. 2007.

[15] Brasil. Secretaria de Educação Fundamental. Parâmetros Curriculares Nacionais: Ciências Naturais. Brasília: Ministério da Educação e Cultura. 1998.

[16] Brasil. Secretaria de Educação Média e Tecnológica. Parâmetros Curriculares Nacionais – Ensino Médio. Parte III: Ciências da Natureza, Matemática e suas tecnologias. Brasilia: Ministério da Educação e Cultura. 1998.

[17] Brasil. Secretaria de Educação Fundamental. Parâmetros Curriculares Nacionais: Meio Ambiente. Brasília: Ministério da Educação e Cultura. 1998.

[18] Miranda EE. A invenção do Brasil. A história da biodiversidade brasileira: nosso país tropical foi um tanto transformado nas mãos dos povoadores e dos povos primitivos. National Geographic Brasil 2007; 86: 60-71. http://viajeaqui.abril.com.br/materias/a-invencao-do-brasil (accessed in 13 January 2013).

[19] Oliveira-Filho AT., Fontes MA. Patterns of Floristic Differentiation among Atlantic Forests in Southeastern Brazil and the Influence of Climate. Biotropica 2000; 32(4b): 793-810.

[20] Freire P. Pedagogia da Autonomia: saberes necessários à prática educativa. São Paulo: Paz e Terra. 25° ed. 1996.

[21] Rosemberg F. Organizações multilaterais, Estado e Políticas de Educação Infantil. Cadernos de Pesquisa 2002; 115:26-63. http://www.scielo.br/scielo.php?script=sci_arttext&pid=S010015742002000100002&lng=pt&nrm=iso (accessed in 15 January 2013).

[22] Tauk-Tornielo, SM. Análise Ambiental: estratégias e ações. Rio Claro: Fundação Salim Farah Maluf/ UNESP; 1995.

[23] Cambuí EVF. Genetic diversity among cultivars of dwarf coconut palm (Cocus nucifera L., var. Nana). MSc. Thesis. Federal University of Sergipe. 2007.

[24] Russo MCO. Cultura Política e Relações de Poder na Região de São Mateus: O papel da Câmara Municipal (1848/1889). MSc. Thesis. Federal University of Espirito Santo. 2007.

[25] Mariath JEA., Vanzela ALL., Kaltchuk-Santos E., De Toni KLG., Andrade CGTJ., Silvério A., Duarte-Silva E., Silva C.R.M., San Martin JA., Nogueira F., Mendes S.P. Embryology of Flowering Plants applied to cytogenetics studies on meiosis. In: Meiosis: Molecular mechanisms and cytogenetic diversity. Rijeka: In Tech; 2012. p.389-410.

[26] Szövényi, P., Ricca, M., Hock, Z., Shaw, JA., Shimizu, K.K., Wagner, A. Selection is no more efficient in haploid than in diploid life stages of an angiosperm and a moss, Molecular Biology and Evolution 2013; 30 (8): 1929-1939.

[27] Taylor T.N., Kerp H.,Hass H. Life history biology of early land plants: Deciphering the gametophyte phase. Proceedings of the National Academy of Sciences 2005; 102: 5892-5897.

[28] Kenrick P., Crane P.R. The origin and early evolution of plants on land. Nature 1997; 389: 33-39.

[29] Bernstein H., Michod R.E. "Evolution of sexual reproduction: Importance of DNA repair, complementation, and variation", The American Naturalist 1981; 117 (4): 537–549.

[30] The Science of Biology. Sinauer Associates. Angiosperm Lyfe cycle. http://www.sumanasinc.com/webcontent/animations/content/angiosperm.html

[31] Gifford E.M., Foster A.S. Morphology and Evolution of Vascular Plants. New York: W. and H. Freeman and Company, 1974.

[32] Aizen MA., Vásquez DP. Flower performance in human-altered habitats. In: Harder LD. And Barrett SCH. Ecology and Evolution of flowers. New York: Oxford Press; 2006. p. 159-180.

[33] Santos RP., Mariath JEA. A single method for fixing, dehydrating and embedding pollen tubes cultivated in vitro for optical and transmission electron microscopy. Biotechnology and Histochemistry 1997; 72: 315-319.

[34] Duarte-Silva E., Rodrigues LR., Mariath JEA. Contradictory results in pollen viability determination of Valeriana scandens L. Gene Conserve 2011; 49: 234-242. www.geneconserve.pro.br (accessed in 26 september 2012).

[35] APG III. Un update of the Angiosperm Phylogeny Group classification for orders and families of flowering plants: APG III. Botanical Journal of Linnean Society 2009; 161 (2): 122-127.

[36] Cornner JK. Ecological genetics of floral evolution. In: Harder LD. And Barrett SCH. Ecology and Evolution of flowers. New York: Oxford Press 2006; 260-277.

[37] O Paraíso de Hello Kitty. [DVD]. Manaus: Sanrio Co. Ltd. 2005.

[38] Chevalérias F., Saltiel E. Ensinar as ciências na escola: da educação infantil à quarta série. São Carlos: Centro de Divulgação Científica e Cultural (CDCC) – USP; 2005. http://www.cdcc.usp.br/maomassa/livro/livro.html (accessed in 13 January 2013).

[39] Castello Branco OH. Uma cidade à beira do Caminho Novo. Petrópolis: Vozes; 1988.

[40] Fundação Casa de Cabangu. Santos=Dumont. Sumário de uma época. http://www.museusantosdumont.org.br/ (accessed in 4 January 2013).

[41] Hedhly A., Hormaza JI., Herrero M. Global warming and sexual plant reproduction. Trends in Plant Science 2008; 14(1): 30-36.

[42] Duarte-Silva E., Vanzela ALL., Mariath JEA. Developmental and cytogenetic analyses of pollen sterility in Valeriana scandens L. Sexual Plant Reproduction 2010; 23: 105-113.

[43] Langridge, P. Food Security, something to chew on. In: Singh, M. (ed.) Conference proccedings of International Congress of Sexual Plant Reproduction, 2012, Melbourne. Australia: International Association of Plant Reproduction; 2012.

[44] Pinto HS., Zullo Junior J., Assad ED., Evangelista BA., Global Warming and Brazilian Coffee crops. Boletim Sociedade Brasileira de Meteorologia 2007; 31(1): 65-72.

[45] Hedhly A., Hormaza JI., Herrero M. Effect of temperature on pollen tube kinesis and dynamics in sweet cherry Prunus avium. American Journal of Botany 2004; 91(4): 558-564.

[46] Shashidar KS., Kumar A. Effect of Climate Change on Orchids and their Conservation Strategies.The Indian Forester 2009; 135 (8): 1039-1049.

[47] Kaul MLH. Male sterility in higher plants. Monographs on the theoretical and applied genetics. Berlin: Springer; 1988.

[48] Shivanna KR. Pollen biology and biotechnology. EUA: Science Publishers; 2003.

[49] Delph LF., Johannsson MH., Stephenson AG. How environmental factors affect pollen performance: ecological and evolutionary consequences. Ecology 1997; 78: 1632-1639.

[50] Lora J., Herrero M., Hormaza JI. Pollen performance, cell number and physiological state in the early divergent angiosperm Annona cherimola Mill. (Annonaceae) are related to environmental conditions. Sexual Plant Reproduction 2012; 25 (3) 157-167.

[51] Nava GA., Marodin GAB, Santos RP, Paniz R., Bergamashi H., Dalmago GA. Desenvolvimento floral e produção de pessegueiros 'granada' sob distintas condições climáticas. Revista Brasileira de Fruticultura 2011; 33(2): 472-481.

[52] Batygina T. Sexual and asexual processes in reproductive systems of flowering plants. Acta Biologica Cracoviensia Series Botanica 2005; 47(1): 51-60.

[53] Barrett SCH. The evolution of plant sexual diversity. Nature Genetics 2001; 3: 274-284.

[54] http://en.wikipedia.org/wiki/Alternation_of_generations (accessed in 22th August 2013).

http://dx.doi.org/10.5772/56929

[55] http://en.wikipedia.org/wiki/Sporophyte (accessed in 22th August 2013).

[56] http://en.wikipedia.org/wiki/Double_fertilization (accessed in 22th August 2013).

[57] http://www.raft.net/case-for-hands-on-learning (accessed in 22th August 2013).

[58] http://www.le.ac.uk/bl/phh4/prosquash.htm (accessed in 22th August 2013).